CULTURE & NURSING CARE:

A Pocket Guide

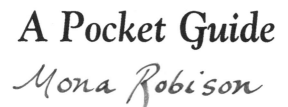

Mona Robison

edited by   Juliene G. Lipson
Suzanne L. Dibble
Pamela A. Minarik

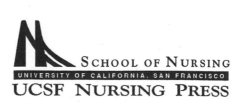

SCHOOL OF NURSING
UNIVERSITY OF CALIFORNIA, SAN FRANCISCO
UCSF NURSING PRESS

Front cover credit:

>Jan Watson (photographer)
>Susan Hayes (weaver)

Graphics:

>Patricia Walsh Design

For information, contact:

>UCSF NURSING PRESS
>School of Nursing
>University of California, San Francisco
>521 Parnassus Avenue
>San Francisco, CA 94143-0608
>U.S.A.
>Phone: (415) 476-2626

ISBN # 0-943671-15-9

Printed in the United States of America

First Printing, 1996

Table of Contents

ACKNOWLEDGEMENTS

————————————

We all wish to thank the chapter authors without whom this book would still be an idea. In addition, we wish to thank the Cultural Diversity Enhancement Committee for their enthusiastic support of this project.

Juliene would like to thank Sue for her help and Chris, Trevor, and Colin for their patience. Sue would like to thank Jeanne, Stan, Maxine, and Marylin for all their love and support. Pamela would like to thank Juliene and Sue for their colleagueship and Lonnie for his love and support.

EDITORS

Juliene G. Lipson, RN, PhD, FAAN is
Professor in the Department of Community
Health Systems, School of Nursing and faculty
in the Medical Anthropology Division of the
Department of Epidemiology and Biostatistics,
School of Medicine at the University of
California, San Francisco. A nurse-anthropolo-
gist, she teaches community health and cross-
cultural nursing and has done research on
Middle Eastern and Afghan immigrants and
refugees since 1982. She is recent recipient of
the 1995 Most Outstanding Paper on Refugee
Issues from the Committee on Refugee Issues,
American Anthropological Association.

Suzanne L. Dibble, RN, DNSc is Associate
Adjunct Professor in the Department of
Physiological Nursing and Director, Research
Support in the Research Center for Symptom
Management at the University of California,
San Francisco. She has authored more than 35
publications and given over 100 presentations
nationally and internationally primarily about
living with chronic illness. She is the
President of the Alpha Eta Chapter of Sigma
Theta Tau and has twice received the presti-
gious ONS/Shering Award for excellence in
cancer nursing research.

Pamela A. Minarik, RN, MS, FAAN is
Associate Professor, Psychiatric Mental Health
Nursing Program at Yale University School of
Nursing and Psychiatric Liaison Clinical
Nurse Specialist at Yale-New Haven Hospital.
Her publications include topics such as ethics
in Japanese health care, communication
skills, cognitive assessment, alternatives to
restraints, imagery in healing, and advanced
practice nursing. She has received the
Margretta M. Styles Award for Excellence in
Nursing presented by Alpha Eta Chapter of
Sigma Theta Tau and the Psychiatric Liaison
Nursing Practice Award presented by the
specialty society.

Culture and Nursing Care: A Pocket Guide

The people of the world can be seen as a tapestry woven of many different strands. Those strands differ in size, shape, color, intensity, age, and place of origin. All strands are integral to the whole; yet each (retains) an individuality that enriches the beauty of the cloth. The tapestry symbolizes the cultural diversity among people. The view of the United States as a "melting pot" has been replaced by the belief that by acknowledging our diversity, greater strength and richness can be created.

It is also important to understand and respect the health care "culture" within which the nurse is practicing. That culture, whether located within the hospital, home, and/or community, is influenced by intersections of forces larger than the individual. For example, capitalism affects the financing of nursing care, especially in a market-driven system such as "managed care." Nursing care is also influenced by shared values about what constitutes ethical professional practice.

We believe it is important to acknowledge another thread in the tapestry: Northern European values and culture. In the United States, these values and culture have had a significant impact on health policy and thus on nursing care. Some Euro-American values and characteristics include: belief in individualism; belief in informed consent; orientation toward clock time; and belief in an order in which God has the most power, followed by men, then women, then children, and then other creatures on earth. There are shared beliefs about the importance of winning, the right to explore and colonize, and the right to defend personal property. There is a commitment to the improvement of the human condition through the use of technology and science. There are also some shared beliefs that illness in the body, mind and spirit can be treated separately.

As with all cultures, these values are neither good nor bad, nor are they exclusive to Euro-Americans. We mention them because of their potential for contributing to cross-cultural misunderstandings in nursing care. For example, a nurse, who believes strongly that an individual has a right and a responsibility to make decisions in his or her own behalf, approaches a patient to teach about a specific treatment plan. If the patient is from a culture in which the family is the decision maker, that patient might nod and smile, expecting the nurse to return when the family is present to discuss the treatment. This type of misunderstanding is common; it can range from a mild miscommunication to a very difficult values conflict about clinical care.

The editors of this book assume that no one person can describe the entire tapestry of human experiences. The processes of this book were to bring together the knowledge of many people about themselves and their strands of the tapestry. The purpose of this book is to offer practicing nurses a snapshot of human diversity.

Preface

We are not providing a cookbook but a set of general guidelines to alert nurses to the similarities as well as differences within and among the groups that comprise the tapestry. We urge readers to use this book as a starting point for individualizing their nursing care.

This book is the result of people of many backgrounds working toward a common goal: the improvement of nursing practice. It is a joint effort of Sigma Theta Tau, Alpha Eta Chapter, the Cultural Diversity Enhancement Committee of the Department of Nursing, University of California at San Francisco Medical Center, the School of Nursing at the University of California, San Francisco (UCSF), the authors, the reviewers, and the editors.

In 1994, the Alpha Eta chapter of Sigma Theta Tau created an ad hoc Long Range Planning Committee that chose to focus on cultural diversity. One outcome of the committee's work was a decision to create a quick reference for use by nurses in caring for patients of cultural/ethnic backgrounds different from theirs. When the Sigma Theta Tau committee discovered <u>Beyond Boundaries</u>, developed by the Cultural Diversity Enhancement Committee, a partnership began.

The idea for the forerunner of <u>Beyond Boundaries</u> originated with Tereza De Paula's master's work in International/Cross-Cultural nursing at UCSF. After graduation in 1990, she and the rest of the Department of Nursing's Cultural Diversity Enhancement Committee created a cultural resource book for UCSF nursing staff. The original manual included chapters about Chinese, Filipino, Korean, Latin, and Vietnamese patients, a list of local ethnic nursing organizations, a list of UCSF interpreter services, and three pages of references. In 1992, Helen Ripple MS, RN, FAAN, then the Director of Nursing, funded the duplication of the manual in a looseleaf format and its dissemination to all acute and ambulatory care units at UCSF. Since the original binder was produced, chapters on Russian, African American, Middle Eastern, Gypsy, and Gay/Lesbian patients have been added.

Selection of groups

The topics for the chapters in this book were selected for inclusion based on size of population (U.S. Census numbering 100,000 or more) or an expressed need from practicing nurses for more information about specific groups in order to improve their patient care (see Appendix A). In a few chapters, several ethnic/immigrant groups have been combined based on their origin from the same world region.

Acknowledgments

In developing their specific chapters, most authors solicited feedback from representatives of their particular cultural group. Some chapters went through an additional review process by outside reviewers and we wish to thank them: Jeanne F. DeJoseph, CNM, PhD, FAAN; Ed Guimaraes, BA; Teresa Juarbe, RN, PhD; Nan Murrell, RN, PhD; Ellen Olshansky, RN, DNSc; LaDonna Osborne, BA; Linda Sawyer, RN, PhD; and Kevin Worth, RN, MS. The following scholars provided population estimates for selected groups: Mehdi Bozorgmehr, PhD; Riffad Hussain, PhD; and Alex Stepick, PhD. We also wish to thank Nancy Evans, James Grout, Fusaye Kato, David Kell, and Sharon Lee and Patricia Struckman for their able assistance with this project.

CULTURALLY COMPETENT NURSING CARE

Juliene G. Lipson

One of many definitions of culture is a system of symbols that is shared, learned, and passed on through generations of a social group. Culture mediates between human beings and chaos; it influences what people perceive and guides people's interactions with each other. It is a process rather than a static entity and it changes over time.

Cultural Competence

Culturally competent nursing care has been defined as being sensitive to issues related to culture, race, gender, sexual orientation, social class, and economic situation, among other factors (Meleis, Isenberg, Koerner, & Stern, 1995). A number of other phrases refer to health care that is tailored to sociocultural characteristics of a particular patient or group: culture-compatible, culturally appropriate, culturally sensitive, culturally responsive, and culturally informed. All of these might refer to such diverse themes as knowledge, interpretation of behavior, attitudes, communication or other skills, nursing roles, and actual interventions. Some critics of the phrase "culturally competent care" argue that it is applied too loosely — nurses cannot be culturally "competent" in a second culture unless they grew up in it or at least are fluent in its language. However, the advantage of "competence" over terms like sensitivity is that it implies not only awareness but also the ability to intervene appropriately and effectively.

Cultural competence in nursing care requires much more than simply acquiring knowledge about another ethnic/cultural group. It is a complex combination of knowledge, attitudes, and skills (Campinha-Bacote, 1994; Lipson, 1998). For example, attitudes are affected by cross-cultural experience and personal attributes such as flexibility, empathy, and language facility. Skills include cross-cultural communication, cultural assessment, cultural interpretation, and intervention. However, this guidebook emphasizes knowledge. It is meant to sensitize nurses to cultural variation, encourage the asking of questions, and stimulate learning about how a patient identifies with and expresses his/her cultural background. Developing further skills such as cultural interpretation or intervention requires additional experience and practice.

Cultural Perspective

A cultural perspective in nursing care includes three interacting viewpoints -- objective, subjective, and the context of the cross-cultural encounter (Lipson & Steiger, 1996). From the nurse's perspective, the objective component focuses on the patient, family, and

1

community's cultural and social characteristics, including communication patterns and world view. The subjective perspective emphasizes the nurse's personal and cultural characteristics. One cannot provide culturally competent nursing care in the absence of self-awareness; nurses need to acknowledge their own values, beliefs, and communication style in order to understand what they contribute to cross-cultural communication. Such awareness can reveal communication barriers based on ethnocentrism or bias toward a particular ethnic, religious, or political group. Discovering one's own cultural baggage requires effort and experience, however, such as reflecting on in-depth encounters with people from different cultural backgrounds.

The context includes the broader cultural, socioeconomic, and political influences on the health care system and their effects on patients and nurses. The context also includes the immediate environment of a cross-cultural care encounter which influences how people interpret what is going on and what they express about themselves. For example, home or community health nursing affords ample opportunity for a good cultural assessment, while time constraints limit such assessment in emergency or critical care settings.

Importance, Limitations and Hazards of Information

By itself, information about a specific cultural/ethnic group does not make for culturally competent care, but neither can good care be provided in its absence. Many nurses believe that one does not need to know about a patient's culture to provide good nursing care; good clinical skills and interpersonal sensitivity are enough. However, we believe that nurses must know something about their patients' sociocultural backgrounds. It is too easy to inadvertently insult a patient when nurses act only on what they feel is correct, which is usually based only on their own values and education.

Cultural information by itself can interfere with care if nurses use it in a cookbook manner and attempt to apply cultural "facts" indiscriminantly to a patient of a particular ethnic group. Cultural information can lead to stereotyping patients, particularly by nurses who lack self-awareness, are ethnocentric, or who fail to recognize variability within any cultural group. Stereotyping differs from generalizing. When stereotyping, one makes an assumption about a person based on group membership without bothering to learn whether or not the individual in question fits that assumption. In contrast, generalizing begins with an assumption about a group but leads to seeking further information about whether the assumption fits the individual. Thus, it is important to learn whether people consider themselves typical or different from others in their cultural group, because age, education, and individual personality influence how individuals express their culture. Because stereotyping comes from jumping to conclusions based on insufficient data or experience with a cultural group, it is useful to suspend judgment as long as possible. However, the paradox is that the more one learns about a different cultural group, the more one realizes how much more there is to learn (Lipson & Steiger, 1996).

Cultural Assessment

A thorough cultural assessment can take many hours, but nurses rarely have that luxury. We believe that, at a minimum, the following list must be included in cultural assessment of any patient (Lipson & Meleis, 1985). The chapters that follow provide information on many other topics relevant to nursing care which could be asked about or observed.

* Where was the patient born? If an immigrant, how long has the patient lived in this country?

* What is the patient's ethnic affiliation and how strong is the patient's ethnic identity?

* Who are the patient's major support people: family members, friends? Does the patient live in an ethnic community?

* What are the primary and secondary languages, speaking and reading ability?

* How would you characterize the nonverbal communication style?

* What is the patient's religion, its importance in daily life, and current practices?

* What are the patient's food preferences and prohibitions?

* What is the patient's economic situation, and is the income adequate to meet the needs of the patient and family?

* What are the health and illness beliefs and practices?

* What are customs and beliefs around such transitions as birth, illness, and death?

Communication and Interpreters

Language differences pose a barrier to even the most basic cultural assessment. Family members pressed into service as interpreters may be unable to assist health care providers because of role conflicts or lack of medical vocabulary. They often base their messages to both patient and provider on their own perception of the situation and may withhold vital information because it may embarrass their family member. Even a bilingual friend, community member or agency employee may be ineffective when untrained, or when not used appropriately by the health provider. We suggest the following when working with an interpreter (adapted from Randall-David, 1989, p. 32):

* Be patient. An interpreted interview may take more than twice as long as an ordinary intechange because careful interpretation often requires long, explanatory phrases.

* Before the session, meet with the interpreter to explain the purpose of the session.

* Encourage the interpreter to meet with the patient before the session to learn about educational level and attitudes toward health and health care to determine the depth and type of information and explanation needed.

* Speak in short units of speech. Do not use long, involved sentences or paragraphs or complex discussions of more than one topic in a single session.

* Use simple language. Avoid technical terminology, abbreviations, professional jargon, colloquialisms, abstractions, idiomatic expressions, slang, and metaphors.

* Encourage translation of the patient's own words as much as possible rather than paraphrasing in professional jargon. The patient's own words provide a better sense of ideas and emotional state.

* Encourage the interpreter to refrain from inserting his or her own ideas or interpretations, or omitting information.

* Check the patient's understanding and the accuracy of the translation by asking him or her to repeat the message or instructions in his or her own words, facilitated by the interpreter.

* During the interaction, look at and speak directly to the patient, not the interpreter.

* Listen to the patient, watching such nonverbal communication as facial expressions, voice intonations, and body movements to learn about emotion associated with the topic.

Even when nurse and patient speak the same language, communication may be hampered by different values or beliefs. Nonverbal differences or regional or ethnic dialects can inhibit mutual understanding.

Communication variations include:

Conversational style and pacing. Silence may indicate respect or acknowledgment that the listener has heard the speaker; in cultures in which a direct "no" is considered rude, silence may mean no. Style of conversation varies between blunt and to the point, and indirect answers, or providing information through stories. A loud voice or a repetitive statement may mean anger or simply emphasis.

Personal space. Cultural patterning often creates erroneous assumptions about individual personalities. People react to others based on their own cultures, rarely recognizing that cultural conceptions of personal space differ. For example, someone may be perceived as aggressive for standing "too close" or as "distant" for backing off when approached.

Eye contact. Culturally appropriate eye contact may vary from intense to fleeting. Avoiding direct eye contact may be a sign of respect, an effort to refrain from invading someone's privacy, or an appropriate behavior between men and women. Cultural differences are easily misinterpreted as negative personality characteristics.

Touch. Every culture has norms about how people should touch each other and in what situation touching is appropriate. For example, there are cultural prohibitions on touching certain parts of the body, e.g., the head among some Southeast Asians, or touching the feet before touching the head. In some groups, physical contact (greeting with an embrace, walking hand-in-hand) with the same gender is more appropriate than with an unrelated person of the opposite gender. In nursing care, examination of the genitals by someone of the opposite gender is a particular problem. Even discussing the topic of reproduction may be acutely embarrassing in some cultural groups.

Time orientation. In some cultures, life is paced according to clock time which is valued over personal or subjective time. In others, involvement with people and completion of interpersonal encounters is more valued than being "on time."

In summary, this chapter outlined a framework for knowledge to enhance culturally competent care, with emphasis on intercultural differences. However, nurses cannot provide good care without assessing both

cultural group patterns and individual and group
variation within a cultural group, which is the emphasis
in the next chapter.

Selected References

Campinha-Bacote, J. (1994). Cultural competence in
psychiatric mental health nursing: A conceptual model.
Nursing Clinics of North America, 29(1), 1-8.

Lipson, J. (1988). The cultural perspective in nursing
education. *Practicing Anthropology, 10*(2), 4-5.

Lipson, J.G., & Meleis, A.I. (1985). Culturally appropriate care: The case of immigrants. *Topics in Clinical
Nursing, 7*(3), 48-56.

Lipson, J.G., & Steiger, N.J. (1996). *Self-care nursing in
multi-cultural context.* Sage Publications.

Meleis, A., Isenberg, M., Koerner, J., & Stern, P. (1995).
*Diversity, marginalization, and culturally competent health
care: Issues in knowledge development.* Washington, DC:
American Academy of Nursing.

Randall-David, E. (1989). *Strategies for working with culturally diverse communities and clients.* Bethesda, MD:
Association for the Care of Children's Health.

DIVERSITY ISSUES

Juliene G. Lipson

Diversity is part of the fabric of North American social life. References to diversity, with all its various meanings, permeate the media as well as the popular and academic literature. This chapter emphasizes sources of diversity that must be considered within each of the racial/ethnic groups covered in the following chapters, and indeed, in any work that describes health beliefs and practices of specific ethnic, racial, or immigrant groups.

Migration: Immigrants and Refugees

Except for American Indians, the U.S. was populated by immigrants from all parts of the world who arrived during different eras. Some groups did not leave their country by choice. Others did not specifically choose to resettle in the U.S., for example, some refugees cared much more about a safe haven than which country offered that refuge. Some had no choice about where they settled, such as Africans who, for several centuries, were captured by slave traders and sold into slavery in various parts of the world. Early in the 17th Century, most Africans were taken to the West Indies and Brazil; they were first sold into slavery in the Virginia colony in 1619.

In considering the health and adjustment of immigrants and refugees, it is important to consider why they left their home country and what drew them to the United States. The U.S. Immigration and Naturalization Service (INS) defines an immigrant as a "nonresident alien admitted for permanent residence." A refugee is a person who is admitted outside normal quota restrictions based on a well founded fear of persecution because of race, religion, nationality, social group, or political opinion. An asylum-seeker is a person who comes to the U.S. applying for refugee status. Undocumented persons (the term we prefer to "illegal aliens") are entrants who do not possess documents allowing them to legally reside in the U.S.

Migration within North America should also be considered. For example, some groups have been forced to relocate, such as the Japanese who experienced internment during World War II and the American Indians who were pushed off their ancestral lands. A radical change in environment is stressful when undertaken for any reason, but perhaps more so because of economic or social necessity, such as farmworkers who migrate to follow the crops or African Americans who leave the rural south to find work in northern cities.

Ethnic/Racial Groups

People often confuse the terms race and ethnicity. Race refers to human biological variation, but the original categories, Caucasoid, Negroid, and Mongoloid, have expanded into multiple racial groups differentiated by blood group and DNA. Racial mixing has given the concept of race little biological significance. But "race" is socially and politically significant because of racism, which is "an oppressive system of racial relations, justified by ideology, in which one racial group benefits from dominating another and defines itself and others through this domination" (Krieger, et al., 1993). Epidemiology also links race to increased disease risks, e.g., increased rates of hypertension and low birth weight among African Americans. However, it is likely that the social context of racism or poverty is as much to blame for higher risks as biology, because these factors expose people to economic and environmental risks and influence interpersonal experiences.

Ethnicity refers to a socially, culturally, and politically constructed group of individuals that holds a common set of characteristics not shared by others with whom its members come in contact. These typically include but are not limited to common ancestry, a sense of historical continuity, common language, religion, and interactions with people of the same group. Ethnic identity is a sense of peoplehood, a consciously shared system of beliefs, values, loyalties, and practices that demonstrates identification with a distinctive group. Some people demonstrate their ethnic identity through a symbolic aspect of culture, such as language or clothing, e.g., Black English, Muslim women's head scarves, or Euro-American three-piece suits. In any ethnic group, individuals vary in the strength of their ethnic identity. In addition, ethnic identity is not static; the social, political, historical, and interpersonal situation may influence how strongly someone expresses his or her ethnic identity. For example, people may have felt and expressed their Jewish identity more or less strongly during periods of anti-Semitism or during residence in New York versus Los Angeles. Religion, often related to ethnicity, is addressed in Appendix B.

Socioeconomic Status (SES) and Social Class

Socioeconomic status (SES) is related to income, education, and occupation. Within any ethnic/racial group, one must assess SES because it may well be a stronger influence on health and access to care than cultural factors. For example, many studies show that poverty is a stronger influence on health and use of health care than ethnic group (Williams & Collins, 1995). Poverty imposes such environmental risk factors as poor or no housing, high lead levels, exposure to industrial toxins, limited access to green open space, and social risk factors such as isolation, gangs, drug traffic, and poor schools. Residents of the U.S. with an annual income below the poverty level have a death rate several times higher than those with an income at or above the median.

Social class origin in the U.S. has relatively less influence on lifestyle, values, behavior, and social relationships than it does in most other countries. Nurses need to consider that among many immigrants and refugees social class is a very powerful determinant of how people relate to each other and differences are played out in health care situations. However, acculturated and educated middle-class immigrants across national groups tend to have more in common with each other and the dominant society than they do with new or less financially fortunate people from their home country.

Sexual Orientation

Variations in sexual orientation also cross ethnic, racial, and socioeconomic groups; thus nurses need to include sexual orientation in assessment of a person in any cultural group. In some areas of the U.S., gay and lesbian subcultures are rich and visible, while in other areas social stigmatizing keeps people closeted. However, nurses often inadvertently offend their gay and lesbian patients by assuming that they are heterosexual instead of routinely asking, "If you are sexual with others, are they men, women, or both?" Nurses may miss important data as well as an opportunity to communicate a nonjudgmental attitude.

Disability

"Abilities" are distributed throughout all populations. For example, there are various skill levels in language or mathematics. Some people with physical or mental health variations are frequently labeled "disabled." Disability, like sexual orientation and race, is regarded variously, depending on the social context in which the individual lives and interacts. Like others whose appearance or behavior differs from the dominant culture, people with disabilities are often stigmatized, discriminated against, infantilized, or seen only in terms of their disabilities.

Cultural variation in perception of impairment relates to the cultural group's conceptions of personhood, identity, and value. Euro-American values of equality and individual ability as a source of social identity shape a concept of disability that may not be applicable in other groups (Ingstad & Whyte, 1995). If, for example, a group perceives that to be a "person," one must be part of a family and have children, and holds those characteristics to be more valuable than work capacity or appearance, then physical or mental impairment may not be as important. It should be noted, however, that in the U.S., people with impairments are legally entitled to the same rights as others and expected to be integrated in the wider society. However, it is also true that "disability" is treated as unspeakable and invisible, e.g., children are taught not to stare at or mention the impairments of the people they meet (Ingstad & Whyte, 1995).

In summary, every cultural group includes considerable variation. In assessing any patient, we must consider such variables as reason for immigration and length of time in the U.S., the social context of bias or racism, strength of ethnic identity, socioeconomic status, sexual orientation, and disability. The intersection of these variables provides experiences unique to each person, experiences which are also interpreted through his or her own personality and resources. The following chapters should not be used as blueprints for patient characteristics, but to alert health providers to potential factors that need to be assessed as a basis for providing good care. We need to trust that our patients are the experts on their lives, culture, and experiences, and if we ask with respect and genuine desire to learn from them, they will tell us how to care for them.

Selected References

Ingstad, B., & Whyte, S.R. (1995). Disability and culture: An overview. In B. Ingstad & S. Whyte (Eds.), *Disability and culture* (pp. 3-32). Berkeley, CA: University of California Press.

Krieger, N., Rowley, D., Herman, A., Avery, B., & Phillips, M. (1993). Racism, sexism, and social class: Implications for studies of health, disease, and well-being. *American Journal of Preventive Medicine, 9* (suppl. 6), 82-122.

Williams, D., & Collins, C. (1995). US socioeconomic and racial differences in health: Patterns and explanations. *Annual Review of Sociology, 21*, 349-387.

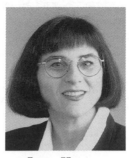

Josea Kramer

Cultural/Ethnic Identity

*   **Preferred term**. People refer to themselves by tribal name (e.g., Sioux, Lakota, Navajo, Cherokee). When referring to all tribes, older adults strongly prefer "American Indians" to "Native Americans." There are more than 500 federally recognized tribes, nations, bands, and native villages and an additional 200 native societies which do not benefit from federal recognition.
*   **History of migration.** American Indian societies had rights to all land now in the U.S. and slowly lost communal rights to all but areas specifically designated as federal or state reservations, rancherías, or native villages. Following World War II, federal policy promoted resettlement in urban areas where the majority of American Indians now live.
*   **Map page.** *See Appendix A, p. 4.*

Communication

*   **Major language and dialects.** Most speak English. American Indians often use anecdotes or metaphors to discuss a situation. Telling about a neighbor who became ill may signal that patient feels similarly. Verbal discourse may be carefully constructed to provide precise meaning through examples, metaphors, etc; do not interrupt speaker. Long pauses are part of conversation. One hundred fifty indigenous languages continue to be spoken; however, do not ask, "Do you have an Indian name?" or "Will you say something in Indian?"
*   **Literacy assessment.** If vocabulary is limited, interpreter (including English) may be needed. At least 56% are high school

graduates (versus all races: 67%)
according to 1990 U.S. census.

* **Nonverbal communication.** Respect communicated by avoiding eye contact; keeping respectful distance recommended.

* **Use of interpreters.** Use mature person, not child, to interpret; prefer same gender. Whether communicating in English or through bilingual interpreter, be sure to indicate if statement based on fact or probability because that information may be part of grammar of some American Indian languages as well as Indian-English. Clinician may benefit from post-hoc translation of what was said, meant, and decided. Use of formal process to interpret information may increase confidence for both patient and clinician, and affirms importance to clinician of having clear understanding (listening highly valued cultural skill).

* **Greetings.** Light touch handshake. Do not refer to men as chiefs or women as squaws.

* **Tone of voice.** Tone expresses urgency; when imperative command required, be direct, emphatic, clear, and calm. In making request, explain why it is needed. Loudness associated with aggression. Requests made in personable and polite manner are appreciated. Humor, self-humor, or willingness to be teased establishes comfortable and positive atmosphere.

* **Orientation toward time.** Present orientation explained as "Indian time," which is flexible and conflicts with rigidly timed appointment schedules. When asking question that requires more than yes or no answer, be patient; expect careful consideration before answering. Rushing an elder considered rude and very disrespectful.

* **Consents.** To obtain consent, have conversation with patient explaining procedure and everyone's role, including role of patient (or family). In asking for signed consent, ask if patient aware that procedure might be needed to achieve better understanding of health problem. Ask if patient needs to consult anyone before consenting; indicate that would be OK. Some individuals may be unwilling to sign written consents based on political and personal history of documents being misused.

Many clinicians note they have not been successful in having advance directives signed, but have achieved an understanding with American Indian clients of preference for natural processes. Overly structured consent processes may give American Indian families impression that they are not being heard, or provider believes they are not competent.

* **Privacy.** Value placed on personal autonomy makes it unlikely that problems of family or friends will be freely discussed. However, illness may be seen as family matter, and immediate extended family may expect to be told condition of patient, test results, prognosis, etc. Names of deceased may be avoided, but relationship term (e.g., sister) can be used.

* **Serious or terminal illness.** Who, how, what, when to discuss prognosis varies with tribe. Some cultures prefer not to openly discuss terminal status and DNR (Do Not Resuscitate) codes because negative thoughts might hasten inevitable loss. Other cultures use information to make appropriate preparations. Clinicians may wish to suggest family meeting to discuss condition and course of treatment.

Activities of Daily Living

* **Modesty.** American Indians modest but not prudish. Offer women gown and robe, and offer men trousers and robe.

* **Skin care.** Varies with individual, so ask.

* **Hair care.** Hair cutting may be associated with health or mourning of a loved one. If procedures require cutting/shaving hair, give extra care to family concerns, and ask if hair needs to be returned to patient or family. If traditional hair style worn, ask how to care for hair and who will arrange hair; allow access to family members who will provide this care. Other customs vary by tribe and include collection of hair from brush, avoidance of touching hair while pregnant, and ritual washing. Family may wish to ceremonially wash hair of very ill patient, including infants.

* **Nail care.** Customs vary. Navajo may take care to collect nail parings.

* **Toileting.** If there are unusual fixtures in hospital bathroom, explain their

purpose. Modesty inconsistent with use of bedpan.

* **Special clothing or amulets.** If medicine bag worn, every effort should be made not to remove it. If removal required, allow patient or family to handle, keep it close to person, in view, and replace as soon as possible. Do NOT casually move, examine, or admire medicine bag.

* **Self-care.** Be sure to tell patient (and/or family) of hospital amenities including library, magazine rack, radio or TV, cafeteria, vending machines, meal schedule, and how to get extra food or fluids if needed. Self-care and self-healing with informal assistance expected at home. Often family may also provide care in hospital.

Food Practices

* **Usual meal pattern.** Light breakfast. Number of meals per day varies with social and other activities, though three meals/day have become norm. Hospitality and respect involve sharing food; patient may wish to share hospital food with visiting family and friends as well as consume food brought by visitors. If patient has prescribed diet, explain to family that meals are nutritionally sound, and that only hospital food is to be consumed by patient. If prescribed diet is to continue at home, explain to family.

* **Food beliefs and rituals.** When food is blessed (traditional religion or Christianity), many people believe it to be devoid of harmful substance; therefore, nutritional guidance should respect religious choice. For example, people will attend social and religious events for which special foods are prepared. Health educators should be aware that rich stews or soups, "fry bread," or other high fat foods may be served, and balance positive benefits of participation with consequences of occasional consumption of high fat food.

* **Usual diet.** Traditional diets were low in fat with seasonal variability, but high fat diets predominate today and the current Pima diet estimated to be 35-50% fatty foods. Government supplied food commodities and Women Infant Children (WIC) programs provide

many rural reservation and urban Indian families with following staples: sweetened condensed milk, cereal, flour, sugar, cooking oil, dry milk, canned vegetables, and processed cheeses. Indian fried bread, mutton stew, and other rich soups and stews are also common foods.

* **Fluids.** Varies but be sure to tell patients that beverages are available between meals.
* **Food prescriptions.** Health educators have promoted salutary effects of indigenous diet based on lean game, seasonal fruits, and vegetables modified for current availability.

Symptom Management

* **Pain.** Pain generally under-treated in this population. American Indians may complain of pain in general terms such as, "I don't feel so good," or "something doesn't feel right." If patient reports being "uncomfortable" and gets no pain relief, patient unlikely to repeat request for assistance. Patient may complain of pain to trusted family member or visitor who will relay message to health care worker.
* **Dyspnea.** Calmly offer reassurance and inquire as to character of dyspnea. Listen for such subtleties of expression as "The air is heavy; the air's not right" which may be complaints of dyspnea.
* **Nausea/vomiting.** Vomiting may be source of embarrassment.
* **Constipation/diarrhea.** When describing symptoms or accepting treatment, patient is matter-of-fact but modest.
* **Fatigue.** May reflect psychosocial issues as well as physical problems. In general, a high level of activity is maintained in spite of a high level of poor health or functional impairment.
* **Depression.** Depression generally recognized, and despite concerns regarding cultural validity, standard screening tests for depression useful. Reporting of depression may be expressed as cultural metaphor such as having "heart problems," "being out of harmony," or having problems with social or physical universe. Often psychological problems presented as vague physical complaints.
* **Self-care for symptom management.** Traditional medicine may be used first or in combination with Western

biomedicine. Preference for Western medicine varies with disease (e.g., diabetes generally recognized as introduced disease with no indigenous ritual or indigenous pharmacopeia), and individual lifestyle (e.g., traditional or "assimilated"). Self-care and self-healing integral to traditional wellness-oriented health concepts. Hygiene will be performed by patient if at all possible. Those cultures having extended family members in same household may benefit from assistance of other family members. However, individuals may be isolated and without informal help in urban areas.

Birth Rituals/Care of the New Mother/Baby

* **Pregnancy care.** Prenatal care expected, and exchange of ideas on this subject generally appreciated.
* **Labor practices.** Labor practices vary with tribe. Mother or other female kin may be birth attendant in normal delivery. Pain control includes meditation, self-control, or indigenous plants.
* **Role of the laboring woman during birth process.** Stoicism generally encouraged.
* **Role of the father and other family members during birth process.** Varies with cultures. Father may be expected to practice certain ritual avoidances (e.g., hunting, eating meat) immediately following birth, generally until the baby's cord falls off.
* **Vaginal vs. cesarean section.** Vaginal delivery preferred. Cesarean section may be feared, based on history of unwanted sterilizations associated with consent for c-section.
* **Breastfeeding.** Breastfeeding and bottle.
* **Birth recuperation.** Mother and infant rest and stay indoors for 20 days or until cord falls off, depending on custom. Remnant of umbilical cord may have spiritual value. Mother given special strengthening foods.
* **Problems with baby.** In hospital, tell birth mother of child. If mother too ill or too young to make decisions, expect that family will be involved in any decision and let family spokesperson emerge. If newborn not expected to live, family may remain at hospital to conduct naming or other rituals which would have been done at home. If

after family returns home from hospital, infant appears jaundiced or sick, mother and child will return for care. Providers need to remember that Indian babies may have Mongolian (darkly pigmented) spot on their lower back and that this is not bruise from child abuse.

* **Male and female circumcision.** Neither expected.

Death Rituals

* **Preparation.** Clinician may want to suggest family meeting to discuss end-of-life issues. Most American Indian cultures embrace the present. Some tribes avoid contact with the dying. If family wants to be present 24 hours a day, this will include immediate and extended family and close friends. If family feels comfortable and welcome (see Visitors), atmosphere may be jovial with eating, joking, playing games, and singing. Small children also included. Although outcome tacitly recognized, positive attitude maintained, and family may avoid discussing impending death. Strong Hopi cultural value is to maintain positive attitude. Sadness and mourning done in private, away from patient. Patients encouraged and not demoralized by strong negative thoughts. Some may prefer to have an open window, or orient patient's body toward a cardinal direction prior to death. Once person is deceased, family may hug, touch, sing, stay close to the deceased. Wailing, shrieking, and other outward signs of grieving may occur, a startling contrast in demeanor.

* **Home vs. hospital.** Varies with culture. Cultures which avoid contact with deceased may prefer hospital. Decisions may include concerns for comfort and naturalness.

* **Special needs.** Be prepared to support or inquire if family wants to bring in other kinds of healers to attend to spiritual health.

* **Care of body.** Care varies with culture and/or Christian beliefs. Traditional practices include turning and/or flexing body, sweetgrass smoke, or other purification; family (women) may want to prepare and dress the body. Family may choose to stay in room with the deceased for a time and then have individual visita-

tion. Health care personnel should ask if acceptable to prepare the body in the room before individual visits begin. Some families will take the body home the night before burial to be cleansed and dressed, "spend the last night on earth," and for visitation by family and friends. Some families may wish the body to rest at place of death for up to 36 hours when soul is believed to depart. Laguna, for instance, do not permit the body to be prepared by mortuary, and family wraps body for burial. Other cultures avoid contact with deceased and deceased's possessions. Family may wish to have all of deceased's possessions including collected hair or nail parings.

* **Attitudes toward organ donation.** If provider initiates frank and open discussion, be sure to distinguish fact from probability, to invite consultation with family members or others, and to indicate that consent or refusal are equally welcome. Organ donation generally not desired.

* **Attitudes toward autopsy.** Generally autopsy not desired.

Family Relationships

* **Composition/structure.** Cultures vary in kinship structure. Examples are matrilineal clans in which related women form extended family core, patrilineages with direct descent reckoned through father-grandfather, etc. American Indians may try to explain relationship as "my brother Indian way" meaning cousin who has same role relationship to me as sibling. In some cultures, homosexuality accepted as is adoption of cross-gender role activities; other cultures do not tolerate homosexuality or cross-dressing except in ritualized contexts.

* **Decision making.** Varies with kinship structure. Autonomy may be highly valued and should not be assumed that spouse would presume an important decision for his/her partner. Children not expected to impose own wishes on parents' end-of-life decision.

* **Spokesperson.** Generally, individuals speak for themselves, but family member may speak on behalf of person who is ill. Family spokesperson varies with kinship structure and culture. If proxy

has not been delegated and family group asks about patient, give information about condition, treatment options, prognosis; explain that providers need to know family's wishes for care and treatment. Let spokesman emerge. Forcing leadership role or other time constraint may not be productive. Spokesperson may not be decision maker.

* **Gender issues.** Varies with culture. For instance, in matrilineal clans or bands, women (and/or their brothers) may make important decisions. Male roles include ritual to protect family and community well-being.

* **Caring role.** Children and grandchildren often assume role for elders. Caregivers vary with kinship structure.

* **Expectations of and for children.** Children expected to respect their elders, take pride in their Indian culture, develop natural talents while maturing. While autonomy generally valued, "independence" is expected to be tempered by responsibility to the community, family, and tribe. Children not encouraged to seek help outside family.

* **Expectations of and for elders.** Elders respected. Status of "elder" recognized when health or physical activities decline at middle age or when individual takes on new social roles such as counseling, teaching, grandparenting. Self-discipline, self-control, and positive attitude toward living are expected behaviors for elders. Home care preferred. Skilled Nursing Facilities rare on reservations (there are only 10) and, unlike general U.S. population, male residents outnumber female residents two to one.

* **Expectation of visitors.** Common for extended family to visit or hold rituals for critically ill person. However, lack of hospital/SNF visiting behaviors have been described for Alaskan Natives and Apache when most likely outcome is death. Whether American Indian visitors feel welcome visiting in hospital setting depends on number of social, cultural, political, and historical factors. Past conflicts may be reflected in hostility toward providers, just as past cooperation may be reflected in genial relationships. As might be expected, family attitudes also vary with circum-

stances for hospital admission
(e.g., condition considered "natural"
part of aging versus unexpected,
violent trauma).

Spiritual/Religious Orientation

* **Primary religious/spiritual affiliation.**
Depends on individual, may be traditional and/or Christian denominations.
Do not expect American Indian
patients to openly discuss traditional
religion. In this last century, Congress
passed legislation to ban traditional
religion which remained in effect until
1979 Indian Freedom of Religion Act.
Despite this law, traditional practice
continues to be prosecuted in federal
court jurisdictions when prayer objects
are eagle feathers or the sacrament
is peyote.

* **Usual religious/spiritual practices.** Depends
on individual and varies with tribe.

* **Use of spiritual healing/healers.** Depends on
individual. May be combined with
Western medicine to promote integra-
tion of healing mind and body. Discuss
with healer how staff can be helpful,
this may include having no staff present and no interruptions of ritual. If
ritual objects, such as feathers, prayer
staff, etc., present, do not casually
admire, examine, or move these sacred
items. If necessary, ask permission for
them to be moved.

Illness Beliefs

* **Causes of physical illness.** Varies with individual adherence to traditional/culture or
Western biomedicine. Navajo traditions may relate physical illness to vio-
lations of social proscriptive behaviors

* **Causes of mental illness.** Mental illness a
culturally specific concept. Beliefs
about cause may include ghosts,
breaking taboos, or loss of harmony
with environment.

* **Causes of genetic defects.** Varies with individual belief in traditional culture or
Western biomedicine. In Navajo,
genetic defect may be
caused by parental violation of
social proscription.

* **Sick role.** Be sick, quiet, and stoic.

* **Home and folk remedies.** Roots and herbs
used for common maladies (coughs,
stomach aches, diarrhea). Some tribes
use purification through sweat lodges.

Lack of trust makes people unwilling to describe practices to strangers.

* **Acceptance of procedures.** Invasive procedures last resort. Patient may be skeptical of procedures but will allow treatment if needed.
* **Care seeking.** Distinction may be made between indigenous health problem requiring native healer and/or practice and Western disease requiring other medical care. Traditional medicine behavior-oriented, holistic, wellness-oriented, and uses visionary diagnosis, in contrast to Western medicine's complaint orientation, organ specificity, illness orientation, and technical diagnostics. Both approaches may be used simultaneously and are considered complementary.

Health Practices

* **Concept of health.** Traditional health beliefs holistic and wellness oriented.
* **Health promotion and prevention.** Traditional health practices include physical stamina (running, aerobic exercise for rituals), relaxation (medication), cleansing (sweats), self-sufficiency, and harmonious living. Participation in relgious ceremonies and prayer promotes health of self and family.
* **Screening.** Those subscribing to Western medicine may desire health screening; however, those practicing traditional medicine, which does not recognize "silent disease," may be reluctant unless efforts are made to explain the value of screening.

Selected References

Garrett, J. T. (1991). Indian health: Values, beliefs, practices. *Minority aging: Essential curricular content for selected health and allied health professions* (DHHS Publication No. HRS-P-DV 90-4, pp. 179-191). Washington, DC: VSGPO.

Hepburn, K., & Reed, R. (1995). Ethical and clinical issues with Native American elders. *Clinics in Geriatric Medicine, 11*(1), 97-111.

Primeaux, M., & Henderson, G. (1981). American Indian patient care. In G. Henderson & M. Primeaux (Eds.), *Transcultural health care* (pp. 239-254). Menlo Park, CA: Addison-Wesley.

Author

B. Josea Kramer, PhD is Associate Director for Education/Evaluation, Geriatric Research Education Clinical Center, Sepulveda VA Medical Center. Over the last 17 years, Dr. Kramer, an anthropologist, has collaborated with American Indian communities on reservations and in urban areas to innovate research and demonstration projects in health and human services. She would like to thank Patricia D. Walsh, M.A. and LaDonna Osborne, B.A. for their extensive input and review of this chapter.

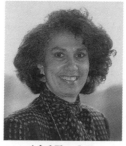

*Afaf Ibrahim
Meleis*

Cultural/Ethnic Identity

*   **Preferred terms.** Identified by region, such as Arab Americans, Middle Eastern Americans—or by country of origin, such as Egyptian Americans or Palestinian Americans. Ask about country of origin; some may identify city (e.g. Ramallah).
*   **History of immigration.**

    Early 1800   Immigrants from Middle East began to arrive.

    1875–1940   First serious wave of immigrants came from what was called Greater Syria.

    Arab Christians came first to Philadelphia World Exhibition and stayed. Mostly Christian men, less educated than later immigrants. Better jobs and higher standard of living drove these immigrants to U.S.

    1940–1970   Second wave driven by political events, wars, and loss of homes. Creation of State of Israel in 1948 marks milestone for increasing Arab immigration to U.S. Moslems arrived during this time as well as large numbers of Egyptians due to political events. Refugees were among this group.

    1970–1990   Third wave of immigrants driven by wars and deteriorating economic and political situation in Egypt. These immigrants were married, better educated, and professionals. More women arrived during second and third waves.

*   **Map page.** *See Appendix C, p. 3.*

Communication

*   **Major language(s) and dialects.** Arabic. Please note, Egyptians also speak "Egyptian-Arabic." Variations exist in

dialects, words and meanings used in different Arab countries. Most Arab Americans understand each other but there are exceptions, such as Yemenis, who tend to speak a more local version of Arabic not widely understood. Although alphabet is very similar, Iranians and Arabs do not understand each other's languages (see chapter on Iranians). All Moslems read same Koran written in Arabic but not all speak Arabic.

* **Literacy assessment.** Arab professionals speak English fluently as do those in small or large businesses. Although they communicate well in everyday language, their language skills may still be limited. Some may assess themselves as speaking English moderately or fluently but still find it difficult to understand language of health professionals and may have difficulty following directions. Also may be too proud to admit not understanding. First ask about their comfort with the English language; comment that they are lucky they speak another language, and then speak slowly, in simple terms and ask for validation of what you said. Since it is insulting to assume lack of language skills among the educated and those who have lived here for a long time, assume fluency until you have data to indicate otherwise. Head nodding and smiles do not always mean comprehension.

    Arabs tend to repeat same information several times if they think others do not understand them. Saying that you understand and repeating will help affirm your understanding.

* **Nonverbal communication.** Expressive, warm other-oriented, shy and modest. May have flat affect to protect others from accessing their inner feelings. More traditional women may be reserved and non-expressive. When they trust and feel accepted, tend to be more expressive. Arabs respect elders and professionals and are reluctant to take up their time. Are comfortable in touching within gender but not between genders. Traditional women may avoid eye contact with non-acquaintances and men.

    Prefer closeness in space and with same sex. When comfortable with others, prefer to be in close proximity to build trusting relationship.

Very polite. Therefore, may not disagree outwardly and may respond in ways that they think others want them to respond.

* **Use of interpreters.** After assessing language skills, inform them of availability of interpreters and give them option of interpretation. Use same sex interpreters whenever possible. Use family members but only same sex family member for translation of sensitive topics related to sex, elimination, marital problems, reproduction, or such highly sensitive diseases as cancer, HIV/AIDS, tuberculosis, or venereal diseases. Note that sometimes family members may edit messages to protect patient.

* **Greetings.** Greet using title and first name. Approach by shaking hands and acknowledge country of origin and something personal about patient or family. Smiling face helps; direct eye contact, even if avoided by patient, is also helpful.

* **Tone of voice.** Loud voice means message is important. Anger usually expressed in high, intense voice by patients and/or family members. Tend to repeat messages for emphasis and for increasing understanding. Arabic a very flowery language with elaborate metaphors; therefore, attempts to translate from Arabic to English increases seeming redundancy. Most tend to express their emotions openly through nonverbal cues and voice, particularly within family. Some of that emotion may be withheld from strangers. May express agreement in front of strangers that does not reflect their true meaning. Tend to protect others from disagreements.

* **Orientation toward time.** More past and present than future orientation, but tend to follow two different time concepts: "on time" kept for official business and more spontaneous time for social and informal gatherings. Human contacts more valued than adhering to clock. If importance of timing emphasized, they are invariably on time.

* **Consents.** Written consent forms may be problematic because verbal consent based on trust is more acceptable mode of

contracting. Dislike listening to all possible complications before procedure. Explain need for written consent, emphasize positive consequences and humanize the process (e.g. when asked for your advice, indicate what you would do for member of your own family).

* **Privacy.** Value modesty and privacy, particularly with strangers. Respect for professionals allows disclosure and loss of privacy. Segregate genders when procedure calls for undressing. Disclosure enhanced by gender matching.

* **Serious or terminal illness.** Family members buffer sick person from knowing whole truth about situation. Confide first in spokesperson of family and consult on best way to approach patient with news. Family prefers to disclose information but may request presence of health professional. If information given in Arabic by family member, no guarantee that seriousness of situation is conveyed. Accommodate family needs for gradual and prolonged disclosure of information.

Activities of Daily Living

* **Modesty.** Very modest. Most need long gown and robe. Drape patient appropriately and carefully, particularly in presence of opposite gender health professionals.

* **Skin care.** Variation by country. Some prefer daily shower; some reluctant to use foreign bathrooms and need careful orientation and support. Some may refuse showers postnatally or during menstruation, believing them to be harmful. Others may not want to shower because of belief that it will undermine their recovery. Orient, explain rationale, and support process. Hospital and its routine intimidating. Careful orientation to all routines will enhance self-care. Some women may wish to use make-up in hospital.

* **Hair care.** Prefer to wash hair weekly. Concerned about catching cold, interference with recovery or management of hair after washing.

* **Nail care.** No particular routines for nail care.

* **Toileting.** Toilet paper not purifying enough. Most prefer to wash after every urination and bowel movement. May insist on using a bidet to wash up after urination and bowel movement. Respect privacy.

* **Special clothing/amulets.** Depends on country of origin. For many women, scarves are important and essential. They like their Koran or Bible handy and may have blue beads or other amulets to ward off evil eye. Even highly educated non-traditional Arabs may believe in evil eye and may keep special amulets during illness.
* **Self-care.** Maintain belief in complete rest and abdication of all responsibilities during illness. Expect family and hospital personnel to take care of them. Energy should be reserved for healing, not expended on self-care. Ask family members to assist. Explain rationale for self-care and its role in patient's recovery and progress.

Food Practices
* **Usual meal pattern.** Three meals per day, largest usually preferred about 2:00 p.m. Do not mix milk and fish, sweet and sour, hot and cold or sweet with meals. Like fruits and desserts. Need to be oriented to meal routines in U.S. and in hospital, particularly if new to this country.
* **Food beliefs and rituals.** Eating important for recovery. Do not give ice with drinks. Hot soup helps recovery.
* **Usual diet.** Vegetables cooked with tomato sauces, chicken, lamb, beef and fish, rice, bread, and pickles. Prefer own food.
* **Fluids.** Water, orange juice as well as other juices, strong black tea with or without milk. Sugar with beverages. Alcohol prohibited among Moslems.
* **Food prohibitions.** Most Moslems do not eat pork, ham, or food cooked in alcohol. Most Christian Arabs eat pork and ham and may consume alcohol. No cold beverages in morning, no icy beverages when sick. Do not offer hot and cold food simultaneously. Will not eat raw fish, rare or medium rare cooked meat; prefer well done meat.
* **Food prescriptions.** Mint teas for abdominal discomfort. Chicken and chicken soups help in recovery. Offering food is associated with nurturing, caring for, accepting and trusting. Sharing of tea, coffee, and chocolates indicates reaching out, trusting, and caring for. Receiving and accepting offers of tea, coffee, or sweets demonstrates accep-

tance and trust. Take time to share a cup of tea or a sweet offering. Ask kitchen for availability of Middle Eastern food; include all wheat pita bread or Syrian bread.

Symptom Management

* **Pain.** (*Wagaa or Allam*) Very expressive about pain, particularly in presence of family members with whom they feel comfortable. Focus is on present pain experience. Pain feared and causes panic when it occurs. Pain to be avoided at all expense. Some may have low pain threshold. Better able to cope with pain if source and prognosis of pain is understood. Tolerance for pain of procedures also high when benefits understood. Differentiate between pain they believe inflicted because staff does not care about protecting them and pain that is inevitable due to procedure or to course of recovery. Express pain metaphorically, using symbols such as fire, iron, knives and rocks. Important for health professional to find out symbols and their meaning. Some patients can respond to numerical pain scale; others cannot. Their response may not reflect reality of pain. Believe injections more effective than pills. Some may perceive intravenous fluids as indication of severity of situation. Explain meaning. Some may be able to manage self medicating. Provide detailed information about differences and advantages and disadvantages. Be prepared to offer advice.

* **Dyspnea.** (*Deeket nafas*) Panic attached to being unable to breathe. Tend to hyperventilate. Need careful coaching about meaning of oxygenation, associated with severity and urgency of situation. May panic more.

* **Nausea/vomiting.** Many will be embarrassed when they vomit. Most do not differentiate between nausea and vomiting; they say "I will vomit" but not "I am nauseated." Some may say "*nefsi ghama aleya*" meaning nausea, but may not translate it as nausea. Vomiting is serious for them because of loss of nutrients. Need to be assured that vomiting not as devastating as seems. Coaching can help them to utilize strategies to prevent nausea and vomiting. Tend to trust that medications may help them

but not as much as other non-invasive strategies.

* **Constipation/diarrhea.** Expect routine BM, and become very distressed if does not occur at specified time. May not volunteer information due to modesty, but will be uncomfortable and distressed. Ask about BM and follow with teaching about lack of significance of routine and time with BM. Constipation prevalent due to low fluid intake (except tea), lack of mobility, and low roughage in American diet. Some may use laxatives for regularity; ask about their use. Will accept medication for diarrhea.

* **Fatigue.** (*Taab, taaban, andy doukha, habtaan*) "Tired, fatigued, dizzy, cannot open my eyes, my blood pressure is low" are all expressions of fatigue. Encourage afternoon nap, ask family members to allow patient to rest. Give them permission to be away from patient so everyone can rest.

* **Depression.** Fatigue, sadness, restlessness, oversleeping, and flat affect are all expressions of depression. Will not acknowledge because emotional well being is believed to be family matter. Encourage patient to discuss; give permission to feel depressed.

* **Self-care for symptom management.** Prefer Western medicine for treatment of symptoms and may use home remedies simultaneously.

Birth Rituals/Care of the New Mother/Baby

* **Pregnancy care.** Some may delay seeing health care provider because they believe normal pregnancies do not need medical attention, or because of expense. Tend to enter health care system late in pregnancy. Much attention given to pregnant woman; encouraged to rest, do minimal work, and eat well. Pregnant women should be given anything they crave. Preparation for birth or for baby not part of most Arab subcultures. Arabs very present-oriented during this process; when it happens, it is dealt with. Need to be encouraged to receive health care, be active, and eat well balanced diet. Need to be assured they can maintain normal routine.

* **Labor practices.** Many myths about labor pains for Arab women. Labor pains

greatly feared. Very expressive during labor with loud noise, moans and groans; some may scream. Father not expected to be present but female family members expected to be present and available. Prefer medications to control pain. Husbands need support as they feel overwhelmed and powerless.

* **Role of laboring woman during birth process.** Active participation in labor a foreign concept to most Arab American women. Tend to tense their muscles and wait for delivery to take place. Hold her hand, fan her, and dry her perspiration. Talk with laboring woman, remind her of her other labor experiences, and that it will soon be over.

* **Role of the father and other family members during birth process.** Father not expected to participate in delivery. Mother, sister, or mother-in-law expected to be present and provide support.

* **Vaginal vs. cesarean section.** Vaginal delivery preferred; cesarean greatly feared.

* **Breastfeeding.** Modernization means giving up breastfeeding. Help mother make decisions and explain the advantages of breastfeeding. Will need help with first baby. May not offer breast because colostrum believed to be harmful to baby. May not request assistance for fear of imposing on staff. Health professional needs to offer assistance.

* **Birth recuperation.** New mother expected to be on complete bed rest after delivery. Mother or sister expected to be in charge of household and family. New mother should eat enriching proteins such as chicken and drink rich fluids made with milk and other ingredients. May take new mother some time to bathe and shower for fear of hurting incisions or introducing infection into uterus. Explain disadvantages of not washing. Very difficult time for first time mother without extended family; needs more understanding, support, and networking.

* **Problems with baby.** Include both mother, father, and aunts or grandparents when discussing baby. They will be taking care of baby.

* **Male and female circumcision.** Male circumcision expected. Some prefer it when

son is about six years old. Others prefer it done in hospital before discharge. Explain rationale for hospital custom. Female circumcision never discussed at birth. If subject comes up, and it does for some, usually arises when a daughter is school age or adolescent. Not based on religious beliefs, but passed on culturally. Arab Americans usually do not attempt to have daughters circumcised. Some may have been circumcised in their home country.

Death Rituals

*   **Preparation.** Arabs do not openly anticipate or grieve for dying person before death. Inform designated head of family privately of death or impending death of patient; allow him to decide how to inform rest of family. Prepare private room for family members to meet and grieve together. In some families, young women barred from being with dying or dead member. Respect wishes of family. Will find it difficult to decide on DNR (Do Not Resuscitate). Family may lose trust in health care system if this option offered.
*   **Home vs. hospital.** Patient who is critically or terminally ill will prefer to die in hospital with family surrounding. Hope that Western medicine may delay death prompts family's preference to die in hospital.
*   **Special needs.** Arab Christians may request minister's visit. Let family initiate visit; provide support. Moslems do not need an Imam to be present. An Imam reads the Koran after the death, not before or during the process of dying. Family's grief is open, loud, and uncontrollable.
*   **Care of the body.** Special rituals followed after death, such as washing the body and all its orifices.
*   **Attitudes toward organ donation.** May not allow organ donation due to respect for burying the body whole and meeting creator with integrity.
*   **Attitudes toward autopsy.** For reasons cited above, autopsy problematic and should be presented with care, allowing family the option of refusing.

Family Relationships

*   **Composition/structure.** Family includes nuclear and extended family. Not

unusual to have within same household uncles, aunts, nephews, nieces, and grandparents. Family-oriented structure. Less tolerant of such alternative family structures as gay and lesbian couples.

* **Decision making.** Families make collective decisions. Extended families also participate in decision making. Father, eldest son, or elderly uncle usually family spokesperson.

* **Spokesperson.** If there is a grandmother, many families defer to her counsel. Physicians expected to make decisions related to care of patient.

* **Gender issues.** Men in immediate family expected to be responsible for logistics of patient transportation, financial arrangements, and funeral plans. Caring for daily needs of patients in or out of hospital usually delegated to women in family.

* **Caring role.** Mothers, grandmothers, sisters, sisters-in-law, or daughters assume caring functions in families. Caring for patients may include preventive self-care and avoiding early ambulation, believing that energy needs to be preserved for healing.

* **Expectations of and for children.** Children are sacred. Families sacrifice money, time, and country of origin to raise children who are well educated and well provided for. Child-rearing based more on negative than positive reinforcement and on what appears to Westerners to be total permissiveness in some areas (roaming in clinics, loud voices, and demanding behaviors) and very strict expectations in other areas (respect for adults, prohibited from speaking back, friendships approved by parents). Parents more strict with girls than boys. Children expected to be obedient with all adults. Some Arab children may have morbid fear of injections and intrusive procedures (used as negative reinforcers in their daily lives). If keeping parent with the child is not helpful, may want to negotiate having parent out of child's room during procedure. Some parents prefer not to be involved in critical procedures.

* **Expectations of and for elders.** Elders respected and expect to be respected. Use title and first name. Some may prefer

to be called mother (*Om*) or father (*Abu*) of eldest son (his first name). Ask family how person is addressed by friends or distant relatives. Children expected to be available at bedside to care for and give support to elderly.

* **Expectations of adults in caring for children and elders.** Extended families, if available, expected to support sick person and family members. Hospital staff expected to be responsible for care of family member. Parents and adult children may need permission to take a rest from caregiving. Absence without urging from staff interpreted as non-caring and non-loving by family.

* **Expectation of visitors.** Social expectations high priority for members of this cultural group. Social visits planned and expected to support grieving or rejoicing families. Reciprocation during mourning and during celebrations an essential part of daily life. Entire families visit sick person and his/her family. Visitors may be treated as family or as acquaintances. Those considered family may be incorporated into care of patient.

Spiritual/Religious Orientation

* **Primary religious/spiritual affiliation.** Early immigrants were Christians, mostly Protestants or Greek Orthodox. Recent immigrants are Moslems and almost exclusively of Sunni branch.

* **Usual religious/spiritual practices.** Prayers usually done in silence. Strict Moslems pray five times a day, and may have to wash before every prayer. When person becomes sick, families may want to pray for him/her. May pray in silence or may prefer another room for privacy. Some patients like to have the Koran or the *Ingeel* (Bible) next to bed or under pillow. Parents may want to pin a blue stone, an evil eye protector, or a hand with five fingers spread onto their children's clothing; These are believed to keep away evil eye.

* **Use of spiritual healing/healers.** Christian Arabs may request visit of Middle Eastern minister. Moslems do not expect an Imam's visit; Imams summoned after death.

Illness Beliefs

* **Causes of physical illness.** Physical illness caused by evil eye, bad luck, stress in family, loss of person or objects, germs, winds and drafts, imbalance in hot and dry and cold and moist, and sudden fears. Among children, deprivations considered cause of illness.

* **Causes of mental illness.** Mental illness caused by sudden fears, pretending to be ill to manipulate family, wrath of God, or God's will. Causes individually focused, not family focused. Could also be caused by loss of country, family, and friends. Mental health care sought only in advanced stages of illness and only after all family and community resources are exhausted.

* **Causes of genetic defects.** Wrath of God, God's will, test of endurance. Religious beliefs call for acceptance but social expectations force isolation from distant family and friends. Disclosure an issue; prefer to "hide" genetically defective family members. Genetic counseling may be refused as believed to defy God's will. Tend to care for children with genetic defects at home and shun institutionalized care.

* **Sick role.** Physically sick individuals treated well. Mentally ill individuals believed to be able to control their illness; therefore may not be treated well by family. Patients expected to assume passive roles in any decisions related to them or others. Patients expect to be pampered.

* **Home and folk remedies.** Western medicine respected and sought after. Home remedies include amulets, sweating, rituals, religious verses, prayers, and well-balanced diets. Folk remedies include herbal teas, camphor ointment, hot chicken soups, and enemas.

* **Acceptance of procedures.** Explain procedures clearly and slowly. De-emphasize potential pain and complications. Seek family member to provide support. Donation of blood may be reserved for loved ones. High acceptance of treatments and procedures expected to cure; low acceptance of complications, viewed as due to negligence or lack of expertise.

* **Care seeking.** Seek early care if no constraints (money, transportation,

babysitting). Delay care for natural conditions such as pregnancy. Seek immediate care for pain. Prefer seeking care from health professionals who provide personal attention. Only seek care from Western health care systems.

Health Practices

* **Concept of health.** Health defined as gift of God manifested in being able to eat well, meet social obligations, be in good mood, have no stressors, have no pain, and have strength. Being overweight associated with health and strength.

* **Health promotion and prevention.** To promote health is to avoid hot-cold, dry-moist shifts, to avoid wind and drafts, to keep warm, well fed and to rest well. Ambulation, self-care, exercise, and hydration need to be explained clearly, stressed often, reinforced constantly. Postoperative activities such as coughing may be avoided for fear of pain. Daily reinforcement of activities and their meaning should be reinforced.

* **Screening.** Arab Americans respect health care systems and providers. Tend to accept any recommended screening if they trust provider's intentions and expertise and if they understand rationale and how it will help them get better.

Selected References

Meleis, A.I. (1981). The Arab American in the health care system. *American Journal of Nursing, 81*, 1180-1183.

Meleis, A.I. (1991). Between two cultures: Identity, roles, and health. *Health Care for Women International, 12*, 365-378.

Meleis, A.I., & Hattar-Pollara, M. (1994). Arab Middle Eastern American women: Stereotyped, invisible but powerful. In D. Adams (Ed.), *Women of color: A cultural diversity health perspective*. Thousand Oaks, CA: Sage Publications.

Meleis, A.I., & Jonsen, A. (1983). Ethical crises and cultural differences. *The Western Journal of Medicine, 138* (6), 889-893.

Meleis, A.I., & Sorrell, L. (1981). Arab American women and their birth experiences. *The American Journal of Maternal Child Nursing, 6*, 171-176.

Author
Afaf I. Meleis, RN, PhD, FAAN is Professor in the School of Nursing at the University of California, San Francisco. Since she immigrated from Egypt 30 years ago, she has conducted research and taught about Arab immigrants in the United States. She is also well known throughout the world for her work with nursing theory.

CHAPTER 5

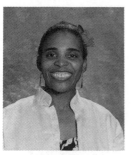
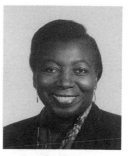

Salamah Locks   *Linda Boateng*

African Americans comprise a very diverse population.
Variations are based on regional, urban, and rural
differences, age, education, and socioeconomic status.

Cultural/Ethnic Identity

*   **Preferred term.** Several terms used depending
    on individual's age and socialization.
    Best to ask what they prefer: colored,
    Negro, black, Afro-American, or
    African American.
*   **History of immigration.** Earliest arrival was of
    20 black indentured servants in
    Jamestown, Virginia in 1619. Some
    eight million slaves were brought to
    U.S. during 18th and 19th centuries.
    African Americans who are descen-
    dants of American slavery are not
    immigrants. Important historical influ-
    ences include emancipation, migration
    from rural areas to cities, and civil
    rights movement. Immigrants from
    Caribbean Islands and parts of
    Africa share some history but
    perceive it differently.
*   **Map page.** *See Appendix A, p. 6*

Communication

*   **Major language and dialects.** English. Some
    traditional dialects spoken in
    Carolinas, Alabama, and Louisiana.
    Black English, a very expressive
    dialect, spoken mainly in inner cities.
    People may switch between Black
    and standard English depending
    on situation.
*   **Literacy assessment.** Ask what level of
    schooling completed. Refusal to sign
    any forms or documents could
    indicate illiteracy rather than just
    being "difficult."
*   **Nonverbal communication.** African
    Americans are affectionate people.

Affection shown by touching, hugging, and being close to friends and family. Maintaining eye contact to show respect and to assess/establish trust. Silence may indicate lack of trust for caregiver.

* **Greetings.** On first meeting, address as Mr. or Mrs. or by professional title and last name. Handshake appropriate.

* **Tone of voice.** When speaking to each other, conversations can get loud and animated. May get agitated or emotional when feeling anxious/frightened.

* **Orientation toward time.** Flexible time frame, not linear. Life issues may take priority over keeping appointments. Primarily present-oriented but varies by individual. Older persons tend to be more punctual and more willing to wait.

* **Consents.** Avoid using medical jargon. Elicit feedback to check understanding. Long history of African Americans being abused as experimental subjects in research may prevent them from readily volunteering for research.

* **Privacy.** Respect privacy; will provide personal information if trust and respect established.

* **Serious or terminal illness.** Best to have family conference or talk with family elder or minister. Patient may have oldest relative selectively reveal poor prognosis.

Activities of Daily Living

* **Modesty.** Respectful approaches are accepted by either gender; may prefer female for both nursing and OB/Gyn care. Muslim women prefer to have their head covered at all times.

* **Skin care.** Daily washing (may choose sink, tub or, shower); skin care important so provide lotions.

* **Hair care.** Hair tends to be naturally dry; hair oils used daily. Braiding, "natural kinky," or permed/relaxed hair styles. Shampoos every 7-10 days but varies.

* **Nail care.** Variable; check individual preferences.

* **Toileting.** Privacy; Muslims may require additional bathing rituals.

* **Special clothing/amulets.** Varies. Muslim women cover hair. Some use prayer beads, wear crosses, etc.

* **Self-care.** Prefer independence if possible; appreciate assistance with difficult to reach areas.

Food Practices

* **Usual meal pattern.** Three meals daily; traditional large meal at late afternoon (supper), frequently practiced on Sundays after church.
* **Food beliefs and rituals.** Prefer cooked foods; pork may not be eaten for religious reasons; greens often seen as essential for good health.
* **Usual diet.** Hearty meals with meat, fish, greens, rice/potatoes, other starches (corn, yams).
* **Fluids.** Cold drinks in quantity: ice water, tea/coffee, sodas.
* **Food prohibitions.** May have religious restrictions (Islamic, Seventh Day Adventists, etc.); otherwise generally no prohibitions.
* **Food prescriptions.** Cooked greens, fresh fruits, red and yellow vegetables for blood/circulation.

Symptom Management

* **Pain.** Expression of pain generally open and public but can vary. Avoid pain medication for fear of addiction. Pain scales helpful to rate discomfort levels.
* **Dyspnea.** "Difficulty catching breath;" acceptance of oxygen, and/or opiates to control dyspnea if explained (fear of addiction is strong).
* **Nausea/vomiting.** Prefer non-pharmacological methods, i.e., ginger ale and soda crackers, teas. With severe symptoms, IV medications welcomed.
* **Constipation/diarrhea.** Open attitude about reporting constipation — "bowels blocked up;" accepts nutritional controls such as fruits, "roughage," especially prunes. Will welcome enema for control of symptoms. Older persons become upset if not moving bowels daily.
* **Fatigue.** Report feeling fatigued or tired; will take sleeping pill to aid in sleeping.
* **Depression.** Seldom acknowledge depression; may view as a "tired" state; accepting of medications to assist with symptoms.
* **Self-care for symptom management.** Home remedies used first; usually role of mother or wife to provide or obtain remedy from a "knowing person."

Birth Rituals/Care of the New Mother/Baby

* **Pregnancy care.** Varies with level of education

and health care knowledge. More than half seek prenatal care after first trimester. Otherwise will seek care when problem perceived, or when care perceived as helpful and accessible.

* **Labor practices.** Expression of pain can be quite open and public; use of medications varies but is not avoided.
* **Role of the laboring woman during birth process.** Active participant. Expects all persons present to do their job, including herself.
* **Role of the father and other family members during birth process.** Varies with health care education of individual(s). Traditionally, only females in attendance.
* **Vaginal vs. cesarean section.** As medically indicated, though vaginal delivery preferred.
* **Breastfeeding.** Varies with level of education and information from other female associates. Most willing to breastfeed if instructed about benefits.
* **Birth recuperation.** Family members care for mother and baby, depending on socioeconomic level and resources. No tub bath/shower or hair washing after birth until cessation of postpartum bleeding; offer sponge baths and provide privacy as needed.
* **Problems with baby.** Rely on older females in family; mother/grandmother.
* **Male and female circumcision.** Many follow Western biomedical tradition of newborn male circumcision.

Death Rituals

* **Preparation.** Report to eldest family member, spouse, or parents; open and public emoting expected but varies.
* **Home vs. hospital.** Varies with individual family situation; frequently care for dying elders at home until death imminent, then bring to hospital. Some believe death in house brings bad luck.
* **Care of the body.** Family members usually want professionals to cleanse and prepare the body. The deceased highly respected; cremation avoided.
* **Attitudes toward organ donation.** Continues to be taboo to donate organs/blood; exceptions for immediate family needs (may hasten own death if donor); some religious restrictions (Jehovah's Witness).

* **Attitudes toward autopsy.** When need explained, most families understand. Physician needs to discuss these issues with family members before patient's death.

Family Relationships

* **Composition/structure.** Nuclear, extended, matriarchal, may include close friends in kin support system. Homosexuality viewed as aberrant but families becoming more tolerant/accepting.
* **Decision making.** In nuclear family, father has final decision making role within household; outside household, egalitarian decision making.
* **Spokesperson.** Father or eldest family member usually spokesperson.
* **Gender issues.** May be separate male and female roles, however very egalitarian.
* **Caring role.** Usually wife or oldest sister or family caretaker, but depends on family structure; sons often care for ailing parents.
* **Expectations of and for children.** Early walking and toileting encouraged. Children expected to help with household chores, attend and complete schooling. Developing talents in sports and music also encouraged to develop socioeconomic base. Discipline and appropriate behavior always emphasized.
* **Expectations of and for elders.** Elders a source of wisdom and demand respect. Often involved in care and raising of grand/great-grandchildren. Independence and appropriate behavior praised.
* **Expectations of adults in caring for children and elders.** Elders cared for in home; children may attend private schools, but are not boarded out. Institutionalization for elders or children for any reason avoided.
* **Expectations of visitors.** Visitors welcome, frequently bring food and/or desserts; family members may/may not sleep at bedside, varies.

Spiritual/Religious Orientation

* **Primary religious/spiritual affiliation.** Baptist, other Protestant sects, Muslim.
* **Usual religious/spiritual practices.** Prayer; visits from minister. Church important African American institution.
* **Use of spiritual healing/healers.** Faith and root healers used in conjunction with biomedical resources. These practices

not readily shared with health care professional. Need to know patient's understanding of illness and beliefs about causes and proper treatment.

Illness Beliefs

* **Causes of physical illness.** Natural causes, improper diet and eating habits; exposure to cold air/winds. Unnatural or supernatural causes: God's punishment for improper behavior or not living according to God's will, work of devil or spell.

* **Causes of mental illness.** Lack of spiritual balance.

* **Causes of genetic defects.** God's will. Some variation with level of education.

* **Sick role.** Illness means that usual roles cannot be fulfilled; based on one's inability to work. Attention from family and relatives expected, but independence maintained.

* **Home and folk remedies.** Teas, herbs, warm medicated compresses to chest for colds; cotton balls in nostrils to protect against cold winds; advice/prescriptions from folk healers who are stable, respected, and powerful resources. Magic or voodoo also used in rural areas.

* **Acceptance of procedures.** Historically skeptical, though with clear explanations, needed surgery accepted.

* **Care seeking.** Both folk and biomedical systems used. Biomedicine highly respected and used for serious illnesses.

Health Practices

* **Concept of health**. Feelings of well-being, able to fulfill role expectations, free of pain and/or excessive stress.

* **Health promotion and prevention.** Proper diet, proper behavior, and exercise in fresh air prescription for maintaining health; protect against excessive cold.

* **Screening.** Open and accepting about new health information; application variable.

Selected References

Capers, C. F. (1985b). Nursing and the Afro-American client. *Topics in Clinical Nursing, 7*(3), 11-2.

Height, D. (1989, July 24). Family and community: Self-help, a black tradition. *The Nation* (pp. 136-138).

Jacobs, C. F. (1990). Healing and prophecy in black spiritual churches: A need for reexamination. *Medical Anthropology, 12*(4), 349-370.

Rooda, L. (1992). Attitudes of nurses toward culturally diverse patients: An examination of the social contact theory. *Journal of National Black Nurses Association, 6*(1), 48-56.

Snow, L. F. (1983). Traditional health beliefs and practices among lower class black Americans. *Western Journal of Medicine, 139*(6), 820-828.

Authors

Salamah Locks, RN, MS, CS is a Clinical Nurse III on a cardiology, cardiothorascic/vascular surgery and telemetry unit at the University of California Medical Center, San Francisco. She is an African American whose greatest inspirator, her mother, was raised by her slaveborn paternal grandmother.

Linda A. Boateng, RN, BSN is a staff nurse at the Post Anesthesia Care Unit at the University of California Medical Center, San Francisco. Born in Kumasi, Ghana, she received her early nursing education at Central Hospital in England and her BSN from Salem State College in Massachusetts.

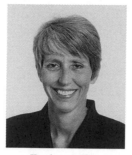

*DeAnne K.
Hilfinger Messias*

Cultural/Ethnic Identity

* **Preferred term.** Brazilian. Although Brazilians
  are Latin Americans, Brazil is culturally and ethnically distinct from
  Hispanic nations and cultures;
  Brazilian immigrants in U.S. often
  resent being classified or identified
  as Hispanics.

  One characteristic of Brazilian
  culture is blending; for example, racial
  and religious mixing and the coexis-
  tence of traditional and modern customs. Racial/ethnic composition of
  Brazilian population results from mixing of native Indian population,
  Portuguese colonizers, and African
  slaves. Other immigrant groups incorporated more recently into Brazilian
  population include other Europeans
  (Italians and Germans), Asians (predominantly Japanese), and Middle
  Easterners (Lebanese and Syrians).
  Brazilians use variety of terms to
  describe resulting racial blends and different shades of skin color (e.g. *pardo*,
  moreno, *mulato*, *caboclo*). Concepts of
  class and social status very strong within Brazilian society.

* **History of immigration.** Prior to 1980, presence of Brazilians in U.S. virtually
  unrecognized. Since mid-1980s, number of both documented and undocumented Brazilians in U.S. has
  increased significantly, although official statistics do not reflect undocumented immigration. Cities with large
  concentrations of Brazilian immigrants
  include New York City, Boston,
  Newark, Philadelphia, Washington,
  D.C., Miami, San Francisco, Los
  Angeles, Austin, Houston, and San
  Antonio. Exodus of Brazilians from
  their country fueled by economic

instability, chronic hyperinflation, underemployment, low wages, and relatively high cost of living. Many Brazilians in U.S. are economic migrants in search of jobs and money. Although many are of middle or lower-middle class origin and often well-educated, in U.S. are frequently employed in low-status service jobs that they would not normally hold in their own country (e.g. domestic service, taxi driver, restaurants, hotels, shoe shine stands, or night clubs). Large numbers of Brazilians also come to U.S. as tourists or students. Some with sufficient economic means come to U.S. specifically seeking specialized medical care (e.g. cancer treatment, cardiac surgery).

* **Map page.** *See Appendix C, p. 5.*

Communication

* **Major language(s) and dialects.** Portuguese.
* **Literacy assessment.** Brazilians vary in level of fluency in English; some recent immigrants may have very limited comprehension and speaking ability. Most likely, however, they will be able to read and write Portuguese. Do not assume that Brazilians speak Spanish as most do not. Spanish rarely studied in Brazil, but some immigrants may have acquired knowledge of Spanish through contact with Hispanic populations in U.S.
* **Nonverbal communication.** Lower class people may avoid direct eye contact with health professionals to show respect. Interpersonal contact generally easy and warm. Personal space quite close. Women may touch each other's clothing while conversing. Men and women might pat shoulder or arm to reassure. Avoid American sign for "OK" (making an "O" with thumb and forefinger), an obscene gesture for Brazilians. "Thumbs up" an appropriate nonverbal sign for "all is well."
* **Use of interpreters.** Recognize limitations of using Spanish speakers as interpreters, since Spanish and Portuguese are distinct languages. Family or friends can serve as translators, but their knowledge or understanding of medical terminology may be limited.
* **Greetings.** Women and youth hug and kiss each other on alternate cheeks, 2 or 3

times. Men hug and energetically pat each other on back. When being introduced to strangers, or in more formal situations, handshakes appropriate, both in greeting and saying good-bye. Persons of lower social class may use the title *doutor/doutora* (doctor) when addressing person of higher status, expression of social deference and not necessarily related to educational degrees or profession.

* **Orientation toward time.** Time subordinate to personal and social relationships. For example, meetings may start when certain people arrive, rather than at appointed hour. In social situations, no one expected to arrive on time.

* **Consents.** Written consent not common practice in Brazil. Medical language of consent forms, and explanation of possible complications and risks may cause concern, confusion, or fear. Patients and family members may be reluctant to question medical professionals about treatment options or to request second opinion.

* **Tone of voice.** Quieter to discuss serious topics.

* **Privacy.** Home and family private matters, but little privacy exists among family members. Being alone often equated with being sad. When dealing with unpleasant or potentially awkward situations, indirect approach considered gracious way of sparing other's feelings and avoiding awkwardness for other person.

* **Serious or terminal illness.** Family members should be consulted before telling patient, as some families will not want patient to "know" or will want diagnosis/prognosis presented to patient in indirect manner.

Activities of Daily Living

* **Modesty.** Women may prefer female caregiver. Young girls and older women tend to be more modest.

* **Skin care.** Hygiene important; shower (or bed bath) daily.

* **Hair care.** Physical appearance valued for both men and women. Men often carry comb and frequently comb hair. Shampoo daily. If bedridden, offer to shampoo hair. May cut hair in accordance with phases of moon.

* **Nail care.** Maintain nails (hands and feet) well manicured; having manicure not just

act of personal care but social encounter (going to beauty parlor).

* **Toileting.** Soap and water peri-wash after BM or urination a common custom; if bedridden, offer daily peri-wash (*higiene íntima*). Women handwash their intimate apparel daily.

* **Special clothing/amulets.** Commonly use crucifix, rosaries, religious medallions, and *figas* (amulet in figure of clenched fist with thumb clasped between forefinger and middle fingers, used to ward off evil). Special colored ribbons tied around wrists or ankles as part of petition to Virgin Mary not removed until they fall off. Spiritists and followers of *Umbanda* (African-Brazilian spirit religion) may prefer white clothing.

* **Self-care.** If patient ambulatory, will perform most self-care; may be assisted by family member. If family not available, offer nursing assistance.

Food Practices

* **Usual meal pattern.** Traditionally, breakfast smallest meal. Main meal eaten at noon and lighter meal taken late in evening. Sandwiches considered "snack" and do not qualify as "meal."

* **Food beliefs and rituals.** Bathing done before meals, because commonly believed that bathing after meal interferes with digestion. Vitamin supplements believed to enhance appetite.

* **Usual diet.** Breakfast usually consists of coffee with hot milk, French bread, and butter. Rice and beans daily staples. Main meal consists of rice, beans, meat, and a vegetable or salad. Evening meal may be similar to lunch or consist of light meal (e.g. soup or hot milk and coffee with bread or cake). Food usually well seasoned; prefer food to be seasoned during preparation and not salted at table.

* **Fluids.** Do not serve ice in water or drinks. Soft drinks often consumed at meals. Preference for glass over plastic drinking cups. Coffee and tea not taken with meals; strong black coffee with sugar (*cafezinho*) taken after meals and mid-morning or mid-afternoon.

* **Food prohibitions.** Certain foods or food combinations thought to have potential to do harm or make one ill (*faz mal*). Cold foods (e.g., ice cream, popsicles, or drinks avoided when person has

cold, sore throat, or respiratory ailment. Milk or milk products not consumed at same time as fruits such as watermelon, mango, pineapple, or lemon.

* **Food prescriptions.** Herbal teas and soups such as chicken and rice soup (*canja*) appropriate for ill person. Bland diets and avoidance of fatty and spicy foods prescribed for cases of "liver dysfunction" (*mal do fígado*).

Symptom Management

* **Pain.** (*Dor*) Generally low threshold for pain; men thought to be less tolerant of pain than women. Will usually describe location and intensity of pain, but not accustomed to using numerical scale. Moaning, crying, or screaming may accompany pain. Women often particularly fearful of pain during childbirth.

* **Dyspnea.** (*Falta de ar*—lack of air) Attributed to both emotional and physical causes. Generally accept oxygen.

* **Nausea/Vomiting.** (Nausea/*vômito*) May be concerned about characteristics of vomitus (e.g., presence of blood). Usually refuse food if nauseated. GI disturbances generally attributed to "liver" problems.

* **Constipation/Diarrhea.** (*Prisão de ventre/ diarréia*) Alterations in bowel function, especially diarrhea, often attributed to food ingestion or intestinal parasites. Homemade oral rehydration solution (*soro caseiro*), medicinal teas, or rice water indicated for diarrhea.

* **Fatigue.** (*Cansaço*—tiredness) Associated with both physical and emotional exhaustion. Management includes bed rest, tonics (*fortificantes*), and increased nutritional intake.

* **Depression.** (*Depressão*—depression; *tristeza*—sadness; *desgosto*—sorrow). May be reluctant to acknowledge depression or seek mental health professional, due to social stigma; reluctance to take psychotropic medications may be related to fear of "addiction." For immigrants, longing for home and family (*saudades*) may be related to depression.

* **Self-care for symptom management.** Whether or not patient is using home remedies or treatments, if medical doctor consulted, generally expect medications to be prescribed. Person who has found folk remedy or

pharmaceutical treatment helpful
may suggest or recommend it to
others; family members and friends
often "share" medications, including
prescription drugs.

Birth Rituals/Care of the New Mother/Baby

* **Pregnancy care.** Family and society give special attention to pregnant women. If
woman has specific desires or cravings
(*desejos*), family will try to satisfy them.
Pregnant woman expected to eat larger
quantities, enough to "feed two." May
solicit ultrasound examination, regardless of medical necessity, to learn
baby's sex.

* **Labor practices.** Male partners generally not
present during labor or delivery. Offer
options for pain relief and anesthesia.

* **Role of the laboring woman during birth
process.** Women often become
less active; some react to pain
with screaming.

* **Role of the father and other family members
during birth process.** Presence of
father in labor and delivery room
often discouraged due to belief that
he may become faint or "not be able
to take it."

* **Vaginal vs. cesarean section.** Woman may
choose cesarean for fear of difficult
birth, for convenience, or due to belief
that vaginal birth following cesarean
not possible or advisable. Rate of
cesarean sections in many private
Brazilian hospitals ranges from 50 to
85%. One cultural meaning of epi-
siotomy is to restore tight vaginal
opening to afford male partner sexual
pleasure.

* **Breastfeeding.** Breastfeeding is socially desired
norm, but belief that breast milk is
"weak" or insufficient in quantity, and
fears of milk "drying up" are common
deterrents to successful breastfeeding.

* **Birth recuperation.** Traditionally, new mother
expected to rest at home, assisted by
her mother, sister, or other family
member. Expected to avoid strenuous
physical activity and outside social
engagements for 40 days following
birth. During this time, baby generally
not taken out in public except for visits to doctor. When in public, infant
often completely covered.

* **Problems with baby.** Both parents should
be informed, preferably by MD. If

mother is single, inform in presence
of family member or friend. Parents
may appear to face infant death with
stoic resignation.

* **Male and female circumcision.** Male circumcision not routinely performed at birth.
In case of phimosis, males circumcised
at older age. No female circumcision.
Baby girls often have ears pierced soon
after birth.

Death Rituals

Recent immigrants may not be familiar with U.S.
hospital and mortuary procedures, so these need to be
carefully explained to family. In Brazil, burial takes place
within 24 hours, and bodies not embalmed. Body prepared at hospital; family and friends maintain constant
vigil by open casket until time of burial. Although traditionally wake held at home, use of funeral chapels at
hospital or cemetery currently more common.

* **Preparation.** Inform family members and offer
to call priest or chaplain.
* **Home vs. hospital.** In cases of acute illnesses,
usual preference is hospital. In chronic
or terminal cases, may prefer home,
but may be reluctant to accept terms
of hospice care (e.g., no therapeutic
measures), because of not wanting to
"give up hope."
* **Special needs.** Family may want to arrange for
extended visitation.
* **Care of the body**. Final good-byes may
involve kissing and caressing the body.
No specific rituals, but family will
choose clothing.
* **Attitudes toward organ donation.** Not a routine or common practice.
* **Attitudes toward autopsy.** Not a routine or
common practice; if medically indicated, provide information and support
for family decision.

Family Relationships

* **Composition/structure.** Close family network
usually includes parents, children,
grandparents, aunts, uncles, cousins,
their respective spouses and siblings,
and may also include godparents
(*padrinhos*). Gays and lesbians included
in regular family activities or
relationships; however, some may not
"formally" disclose their homosexuality
to family, and family in turn never
explicitly acknowledges what is
informally regarded as "common
knowledge." Family is center of social
activities, and also serves as resource

for mutual aid and social and economic assistance. Brazilians have strong sense of family loyalty and of duty to help relatives, and will often prefer to seek help from family rather than professionals or social agencies. Being separated from their traditional family support system often source of stress and sadness for immigrants.

* **Decision making.** Within nuclear family, parents or spouse take decision making role. In extended family, those with more education and/or economic means usually occupy role of family counselor or advisor, as well as providing material support in times of need.

* **Spokesperson.** Parents or spouse.

* **Gender issues.** Traditional families patriarchal. Male, as head of family (*chefe da família*), expected to provide for family's material and economic necessities. Female, as head of house (*dona da casa*), responsible for managing home, even if engaged in outside employment.

* **Caring role.** Women principal caregivers, also main sources of knowledge and expertise regarding home remedies and treatments, particularly older women.

* **Expectations of and for children.** Parental treatment and expectations differ for sons and daughters. Girls in general expected to be more docile, submissive, calm, and interested in school. Boys considered more competitive, given more freedom, and not held to same standards of discipline as girls. Adult children often remain in parents' home until marriage; some remain after marriage. Voluntary childlessness uncommon.

* **Expectations of and for elders.** Elders usually remain in home, and social contacts revolve around family. Adult children expected to provide both economic security and social companionship for parents in old age.

* **Expectations of adults in caring for children and elders.** Family members primary caregivers for both children and elder. Home care preferred to institutionalization or nursing home. Those with economic means will employ nannies or home health aides.

* **Expectation of visitors.** If patient hospitalized, particularly in private room, expected that companion

(*acompanhante*) remain with patient. Family members or close friends may rotate in role of *acompanhante* to assure that someone is with patient. Frequent visits by other friends and family expected.

Spiritual/Religious Orientation

* **Primary religious/spiritual affiliation.** Majority of Brazilians identify themselves as Catholics, but growing number of Evangelicals and Protestants. Other religions include Brazilian Spiritist or *Kardecist*, a systematized doctrine about spirit mediums and spirit world developed by Allan Kardec, 19th century French educator; *Umbanda*, an indigenous Brazilian religion characterized by blending of African and Amerindian spiritism and folk Catholicism; and *Candomblé*, an African-Brazilian spiritist religion.

* **Usual religious/spiritual practices.** Catholic folk practices focus on saints, promises, and pilgrimages. Strong belief in miracles and miracle cures, many of which are attributed to saints by devoted. Spirit mediumship and spiritual healing part of popular Catholic practices and various spiritist religions.

* **Use of spiritual healing/healers.** Brazilians have strong traditions of religious/spiritual healing. Catholic priests called in case of emergencies and for sacrament of the sick. Spiritists practice laying on of hands (*passes*). Blessings and prayers by folk healers (*benzedeiras, curandeiras*) often given in conjunction with herbal remedies.

Illness Beliefs

* **Causes of physical illness.** May be attributed to divine intervention or fate. Acute illnesses often associated with activity, change in temperature, food ingestion, or strong emotion that occurred prior to onset. Common belief that infants and young children can become ill if exposed to bursts of fresh air or wind (*pegar vento*).

* **Causes of mental illness.** Folk syndromes known as *nervos, ataque de nervos*, and *susto* associated with suppression of strong negative emotions such as anger, fear, envy, worry, sadness or grief.

* **Causes of genetic defects.** Common explanation is fatalistic view of "God's will" (*vontade de Deus/Deus quis*). May also be attributed to events occurring during pregnancy (e.g., accidents, emotional shocks) or to defective sperm, sometimes associated with excessive alcohol use. Some parents accept child's genetic or congenital defects, while others harbor strong feelings of guilt or shame.
* **Sick role.** Ill person expected to receive attention and care from others.
* **Home and folk remedies.** Vast array of medicinal herb baths, teas, and remedies, sometimes used in conjunction with special prayers and blessings.
* **Acceptance of procedures.** Often prefer IM and IV injections to other forms of medication. Patient and family may monitor duration and quantity of IV infusions as indication of severity or prognosis of patient's condition.
* **Care seeking.** Often concurrently use different types of treatment, such as homeopathy, acupuncture, medicinal herbs, and spiritual healing, with allopathic medicine. Self-medication with antibiotics and other drugs available over-the-counter in Brazil is common practice, often before seeking health care from professionals. Aware that such drugs are not available without prescription in U.S., immigrants frequently bring supplies of such drugs with them or have them sent from Brazil.

Health Practices

* **Concept of health.** Usually considered absence of pain, suffering, or disease. Health may also be considered divine blessing. Weight gain, in both children and adults, is considered sign of "health."
* **Health promotion and prevention.** Seek medical professionals primarily for treatment of existing illness rather than promotion or prevention.
* **Screening.** May not actively seek screening for conditions when no apparent symptoms. Reluctance to undergo screening may be rooted in fear of uncovering disease or not wanting to face "bad news."

Selected References

Margolis, M. L. (1995). Brazilians and the 1990 United

States census: Immigrants, ethnicity, and the under-count. *Human Organization, 54*(1), 52-59.

Rebhun, L. A. (1994). Swallowing frogs: Anger and illness in Northeast Brazil. *Medical Anthropology Quarterly, 8*(4), 360-382.

Author

DeAnne K. Hilfinger Messias, RN, MS, PhD(c) is a community health nurse and doctoral candidate at the University of California, San Francisco, School of Nursing, studying the migration, work, and health experiences of Brazilian immigrant women. She lived in Brazil for over 20 years, where she was involved in nursing education programs and directed a rural primary health care program on the Amazon River.

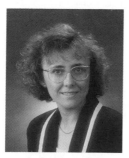

Judith C. Kulig

Cultural/Ethnic Identity
* **Preferred terms.** Khmer—(pronounced Kami).
Sino-Khmer refers to Chinese-Cambodians.
* **History of immigration.**
Before 1970, only few hundred Khmer in U.S.

1975	Well-educated professionals affiliated with American government. Evacuated directly to U.S. due to impending civil war.
1975–1979	Well-educated professionals escaped on their own and after brief stays in Thai refugee camps were resettled in countries such as U.S. and Canada.
1980–1985	Although well-educated individuals and families continued being resettled, larger numbers of rural agrarian individuals and families arrived. Many were widows and orphans due to brutal civil war. Large percentage lacked skills necessary to life in U.S.
1985–present.	Most arrivals sponsored by their families who are now American citizens.

* **Map page.** *See appendix C, p. 6.*

Communication
* **Major language(s) and dialects.** Khmer major dialect but also name of the people. Khmer tribal dialects exist but few speak them. Written language based on Sanskrit from India.
* **Literacy assessment.** Speak slowly with no jargon or idioms. Many elderly Khmer cannot read and write own language. Younger Khmer have lost ability to read and write their language and are more fluent in English.
* **Nonverbal communication.** Inappropriate to touch their heads without permission because some believe the soul is in the head. Silence welcomed and more appropriate than meaningless chatter.

Eye contact acceptable but "polite" women lower their eyes somewhat. Khmer people shy but affectionate to one another and have a small personal space. Considered impolite to disagree—may say yes but not do as expected.

* **Use of interpreters.** Include family members when discussing health condition. Sensitive issues, such as sexuality, should include translator of same gender.

* **Greetings.** *Sompeah*, gesture of both palms brought together with fingers pointed upward, used to greet others. Height of *sompeah* indicates status of individual being greeted. More acculturated greet with handshakes. Terms such as *om* (great aunt or uncle), *pu* (uncle), *miin* (aunt), *baan* (older sibling) used when talking with friends, otherwise *look* (Sir, Mister) or *look srey* (Mrs.) used.

* **Tone of voice.** Quiet tone of voice. Very important to speak softly and be polite

* **Orientation toward time.** Flexible attitude toward time; tardiness for appointments expected. Emphasis on past (remembering ancestors) but also on present because actions today will determine future. Khmer predominantly Buddhists, believe in rebirth. *Samsara* refers to continual birth and death, an important concept.

* **Consents.** Among middle-aged and older Khmer, discomfort with written consents due to Khmer Rouge war in which signed life histories were required from those later executed. Research consents best if verbal only. Ensure accurate translation and understanding for consents for health-related procedures.

* **Privacy.** Saving face important. Trust friends and family members as interpreters. Have respect for authority figures and will discuss some issues but hesitant when discussing sexuality, mental health symptoms, and alternative healing practices.

* **Serious or terminal illness.** Discuss with family first and allow them to discuss with ill family member. Offer to answer questions or clarify concerns.

Activities of Daily Living
* **Modesty.** Very modest, uncomfortable with exposing body. More comfortable wit

care provider of same gender but comfortable with male physicians.

* **Skin care.** Daily showers—infants and children (to age 2 years) "washed down" after each diaper change.

    Young women take considerable time in caring for their skin; make-up extremely important.

* **Hair care.** Wash hair daily. Young people use many hair products. Young women have long hair; after marriage (particularly after first child is born), hair is cut.

* **Nail care.** Men keep nail of right little finger longer than other fingernails. Women meticulous about nail care.

* **Toileting.** Older Khmer more accustomed to squatting; may be uncomfortable with bedpan, urinal, etc.

* **Special clothing/amulets.** Young unmarried women who are menstruating wear a protective string and cloth bag around their waist to prevent "love magic," having love spell placed on them. Adults and children may wear string or chain around neck with amulet containing Buddhist transcription for protection. Do not remove either without permission.

* **Self-care.** Hygiene performed by patient. Family members involved in providing care and bringing food to ill family member.

Food Practices

* **Usual meal pattern.** Rice a staple, eaten at all three meals. Individuals have own bowls and take food from communal bowls.

* **Food beliefs and rituals.** Believe hot/cold properties inherent in food. Rice considered neutral, chicken hot, vegetables cold. Combination of ingredients also determines hot/cold properties. For example, adding coconut cools things down.

* **Usual diet.** Breakfast often chicken soup or noodle dish. Other meals include rice or noodles with fish paste and vegetables. More elaborate meals also prepared, such as pancakes (similar to crepes) with pork, bean sprouts, and fish sauce. Younger Khmer like Western foods.

* **Fluids.** Lactose intolerant; like soy drinks and specially brewed coffee. Do not use ice. Prefer warm tea or water.

* **Food prohibitions.** See Pregnancy care and Birth recuperation.
* **Food prescriptions.** See Pregnancy care.

Symptom Management

* **Pain.** Stoic when in pain, prefer IM or SC injection. Use of tiger balm, medicated tapes placed on painful area, and cupping practice in which penny with birthday size candle is placed on forehead, candle is lit and inverted glass jar placed on top. When jar is removed, dark circle appears on forehead. Believe this practice sucks out pain, used for headaches or other type pain.
* **Dyspnea.** Anxious if cannot breathe. Some Khmer have died from SUNDS (Sudden Unexpected Nocturnal Death Syndrome), inability to breathe plus cardiac symptoms.
* **Nausea/Vomiting.** Will interpret nausea/vomiting as balance problem within gastrointestinal system and likely restrict particular foods. Ask if they feel in balance.
* **Constipation/Diarrhea.** Modesty prevents open discussion of altered bowel habits. Enemas need to be explained carefully.
* **Fatigue.** Fatigue believed related to other symptoms or problems.
* **Depression.** Uncomfortable discussing mental health symptoms. Depression explained as sadness. Western medicine believed "too strong" for their bodies; may decrease medication dosage or not take pills. Older Khmer women attribute memory loss and depression to brutalities of Khmer Rouge war.
* **Self-care for symptom management.** Use alternative healers and healing practices. Often go to Western professionals and Vietnamese or Cambodian physicians simultaneously to receive adequate care.

Birth Rituals/Care of the New Mother/Baby

* **Pregnancy care.** Elderly women give prenatal advice about diet and activities. Uncomfortable with Western approach to prenatal classes. No emphasis on prenatal checkups.

    Pregnant women follow specific activity restrictions (e.g., do not stand in doorway as baby will be stuck in birth canal; do not step over others when pregnant). Pregnant women active. Ingestion of some foods avoided but special foods with coconut sanctioned. Herbal medicines used in last trimester for healthy baby. Sexual intercourse not permitted during last trimester. Vernix caseosa believed to be sperm. During last trimester, herbal medicines prepared for postpartum use.

* **Labor practices.** Walking during labor acceptable. Husband may not choose to be with wife. Her mother or *chomp* (midwife) may assist.

* **Role of the laboring woman during birth process.** Laboring woman should be stoic. Pain relief should be offered.

* **Role of the father and other family members during birth process.** Depends on individual situation. Some laboring women do not want husband present but their mothers are acceptable.

* **Vaginal vs. cesarean section.** Vaginal delivery preferred.

* **Breastfeeding.** Breastfeeding delayed a few days because colostrum believed inappropriate for baby. Bottle feeding believed to imply higher status. Modest when exposing breasts. Reluctant to ask questions about positioning, etc. Baby routinely held down and away from mother; cuddling uncommon. Babies (and adults) not kissed but sniffed to show affection.

* **Birth recuperation.** New mother is to rest for first few weeks with mother or mother-in-law very involved in baby's and mother's care. New mother wears heavy clothing (including scarf and toque) and eats special foods to restore heat lost in birth process. Warm tea and water given. Vegetables ("cold") restricted. Chicken ("hot") acceptable. Herbal medicines ingested 3-4 times daily to restore body heat. Peri-care and cleanliness important, but full body shower may not be taken. Family members and friends of both genders come to see baby and mother. Baby shower held a few weeks after birth, attended by entire families.

* **Problems with baby.** Discuss with father and family and then with new mother. Adequate translation essential. Due to numerous activity restrictions, couple may blame problem on their

own incorrect behavior. Limited
understanding of genetics.
* **Male and female circumcision.**
Neither practiced.

Death Rituals
* **Preparation.** Inform parents or older
children. Encourage them to call
other family members, monks, and
aacha (religious layperson).
* **Home vs. hospital.** For chronic illness, prefer
to die at home so family members
can care for dying person. Feel
comfortable with acutely ill person
dying in hospital.
* **Special needs.** Monks and *aacha* need to be
called to recite prayers. Family members should also be present. Death
faced by family in quiet, passive manner. Incense may be burned.
* **Care of the body.** Family, monks, and *aacha*
may want to wash the body. The body
is shrouded in white cloth. Those in
mourning wear white. Prayers by monk
on night of the death also important;
explain to family about release of the
body. Sorrow a limited phase.
* **Attitudes toward organ donation.** Unlikely
to allow organ donation. Body
cremated. Due to belief in rebirth and
possible better reincarnation, desire
body to be intact.
* **Attitudes toward autopsy.** Unlikely to
agree to autopsy. If essential, careful
explanation needed.

Family Relationships
* **Composition/structure.** Family-oriented. Due
to many losses of family members in
war, fictive kinship practiced (i.e.,
non-biological relatives considered as
kin). Three generations frequently live
in one house. Homosexuality unacceptable. Acceptable for heterosexual
men or women to hold hands with
same gender.
* **Decision making.** Elders key in decision making. Wives "convince" their husbands
about decisions.
* **Spokesperson.** Father, eldest son, or daughter.
* **Gender issues.** Traditional roles common but
some women have worked at a trade
within their home as jewelry sellers,
for example. Men help with domestic
chores and childrearing. Women
expected to be caregivers.

* **Caring role.** Women, particularly elderly, are major caregivers.
* **Expectations of and for children.** Polite, quiet, obedient children are norm. Vocal sounds used to discipline children. Girls' behavior more restricted (e.g., family loses honor if girl loses virginity premaritally). Children expected to attend post-secondary education.
* **Expectations of and for elders.** Elders highly respected; special words of address used. Assist in child care but otherwise will visit or play cards with other elders. Children to take care of their parents. Organized group of Senior Khmer in U.S. assists financially in providing appropriate funeral services.
* **Expectations of adults in caring for children and elders.** Adults, especially women, to care for ill family members in their home until health is restored.
* **Expectation of visitors.** Family members and friends visit at bedside; important that patient not be alone.

Spiritual/Religious Orientation
* **Primary religious/spiritual affiliation.** Predominantly Theravada Buddhist but some have converted to Christianity. Khmer practice syncretism, a blend of Buddhism, Animism, and, sometimes, Christianity.
* **Usual religious/spiritual practices.** Within Buddhism, a number of celebrations throughout year—*Caul Chnam*; Cambodian New Year (April 12 - 13), *Pcom Bun* (celebration similar to Thanksgiving); *Bun Kaʔthən* (celebration to provide for monks)—incorporating religious activities with festive party. Most homes have altar to which food offerings and incense are offered daily. Holy water used by monks and accha. The *accha* always male and performs marriage ceremony as well as healing ceremonies. Inappropriate for women to touch a monk. *Yiey chii* are Buddhist nuns (often postmenopausal) who may live in the *wat* (temple) all year or for specific days each month. Days correlate with moon phases signifying Buddha's birth. At each meal, including weddings, dish of food set for ancestral spirits.
* **Use of spiritual healing/healers.** *Accha* performs elaborate diagnostic activities

and healing ceremonies in person's home. *Krou* are healers specialized in dealing with certain illnesses. *Krous* may visit patient but not disclose to health professionals who they are. *Thump* are evil *Krous* who place spells on people.

Illness Beliefs

* **Causes of physical illness.** Hot/cold imbalance; specific activities (e.g. labor camps in Khmer Rouge takeover have left many Khmer with back and limb problems); *thump* activities; or sins of past life.
* **Causes of mental illness.** Khmer Rouge brutalities.
* **Causes of genetic defects.** Do not understand genetics, blame defects on past sins or parents' indiscretions during pregnancy.
* **Sick role.** Passive role when ill, expect to be cared for. Extra attention given to the ill.
* **Home and folk remedies.** Uncomfortable discussing alternative remedies. Herbal medicines common, Chinese and Indian influence evident in types of herbal medicines used. Herbal medicines, medicated strips of adhesive tape, and activities such as cupping and coining (rubbing anterior and posterior chest wall with a coin in a downward vigorous fashion to diagnosis and treat illness). Coining believed to work by releasing heat.
* **Acceptance of procedures.** Uncomfortable with giving blood or blood specimens due to heat loss. Explain about transfusions, etc. May not accept organ transplants.
* **Care seeking.** Simultaneous use of Western and traditional healing practices. Latter provides psychological comfort.

Health Practices

* **Concept of health.** Being healthy important; seen as being in equilibrium. Health needs to be individually maintained but is influenced by family and community members, e.g., if *thump* intervenes, person can become ill; if young couple engage in premarital sexual intercourse, *meba* (ancestral spirits) can make family members ill.
* **Health promotion and prevention.** Illness seen as preventable. Nutrition

important but not physical activity. Health education should be discussed in culturally appropriate manner (i.e., discuss diabetes diet using Cambodian food).

*   **Screening.** Accustomed to screening for diseases but modesty can be an issue with some types of diagnostic tests. Careful explanations to patient and family always best.

Selected References

Frye, B. (1991). Cultural themes in health-care decision making among Cambodian refugee women. *Journal of Community Health Nursing, 8*(1), 33-44.

Kulig, J. (1995). Cambodian refugees' family planning knowledge and use. *Journal of Advanced Nursing, 22,* 150-157.

Rasbridge, L., & Kulig, J. (1995). Infant feeding among Cambodian refugees. *Maternal Child Nursing, 20*(4), 213-218.

Sargent, C., Marcucci, J., & Elliston, E. (1983). Tigerbones, fire and wine: Maternity care in a Kampuchean refugee community. *Medical Anthropology: Cross Cultural Studies in Health & Illness, 1*(4), 67-79.

Author

Judith C. Kulig, RN, DNSc is an Associate Professor in the School of Nursing and Research Coordinator of the Regional Centre for Health Promotion and Community Studies at the University of Lethbridge, Canada. She has worked as a public health nurse, educator, and researcher with a variety of groups including Khmer, Vietnamese, Central Americans, Navajo, Hopi, and Tsimshian aboriginal groups.

(Salvadorans, Guatemalans, and Nicaraguans)

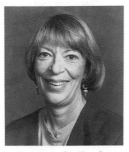

Joyceen S. Boyle

Cultural/Ethnic Identity

* **Preferred term**. Most Central Americans prefer to be addressed with their specific country in mind. Thus, terms such as Guatemalans, Nicaraguans, or Salvadorans are appropriate.
* **History of immigration.** Central Americans have come to U.S. for many years, primarily for economic reasons. Around late 1970s, Guatemala, Nicaragua, and El Salvador experienced considerable political violence with profound effects on all citizens. Consequently, many fled their country of origin to escape devastating circumstances at home. Their legal status in U.S. has often been precarious.
* **Map page.** *See Appendix C, p. 2.*

Communication

* **Major language(s) and dialects.** Spanish is national language of all Central American countries. However, Guatemala has large Mayan population (slightly less than half of all residents are Mayan Indian). There are 18 or more Mayan dialects in use today, and some rural Maya do not speak Spanish. Guatemala also has a Black Carib culture, and El Salvador and Nicaragua have Indian populations, all with distinct languages and dialects.
* **Literacy assessment.** Most Central Americans speak and understand Spanish, except for Mayan Indians who have lived in rural and isolated areas of Guatemala, although most speak some Spanish. Reading and writing of Spanish may be limited. Many Mayan Indians have not had opportunity to attend school and thus may not be able to read or write proficiently. Traditional role of women may be valued over school attendance.

If clients have some proficiency with English, important to speak very slowly and use simple terms and phrases.

* **Nonverbal communication.** Most Central Americans friendly, gracious, hospitable. Mayan women may be very shy. Health professionals respected as are elders and authority figures. In Latin cultures, touching (between members of same sex) is common. Nonverbal gestures frequently used. Do not have same need for personal space as most North Americans.

* **Use of interpreters.** Allow time for interpreter and client/family to get to know one another, if possible. Be sensitive to issues such as gender and age, especially if using family member as interpreter.

* **Greetings.** Central Americans friendly and outgoing; gracious manner expected. Kissing as greeting common between women. Relationships among family members or persons from same geographical location are close and enduring.

* **Tone of voice.** Spanish a rich language, full of intonations and meanings that might be difficult for novice. Central Americans somewhat formal; use formal Spanish rather than informal form.

* **Orientation toward time.** Traditionally, Latin American cultures have different view of time and importance of punctuality than North Americans. Little concern for exact time of day. Lunch can be leisurely with little thought of later appointment. Promptness and concern with schedules not important; Central Americans bewildered by health professionals' impatience or annoyance with those late for appointments.

* **Consents.** Explain procedures very carefully. Central American countries have different legal concepts and procedures than those common in U.S. The concept of Informed Consent or Patients' Rights unfamiliar to many Central Americans with no previous contact with health care system.

* **Privacy.** Central American women, especially Mayan women, may be very shy around strangers such as physicians and nurses. Isolation from extended family members during hospitalizat' may create stress and feelings of

65

vulnerability because it interferes with traditional support systems. Allow family members to be present.

* **Serious or terminal illness.** Consult with father or eldest son before disclosing serious illness to patient. Disclosing prognosis may not be valued in Latin cultures, and family members may choose not to tell patient he/she has terminal illness. Solicit wishes of family members.

Activities of Daily Living

* **Modesty.** Very modest, particularly women. Offer hospital gowns and robes. Screening and reassurance during procedures important. Modesty includes covering legs. Mayan women comfortable breastfeeding babies in public. Many Latin women (and their husbands) may prefer female physician if available.

* **Skin care.** Offer opportunity to bathe or shower daily. Some clients recently arrived in U.S. may prefer not to bathe or shower that frequently.

* **Hair care.** Mayan women may conform to traditional values and not cut their hair but braid it. May cover head with traditional scarf or head covering. Long hair not washed daily.

* **Nail care.** Women from higher socioeconomic levels may seek regular manicures and use nail polish. Because of traditional values, work roles, or religious teachings, other women do not wear nail polish.

* **Toileting.** Privacy important to both men and women when hospitalized. First hospitalization may require orientation to bedpan, urinal, other hospital procedures.

* **Special clothing/amulets.** Traditionally Catholic, although Pentecostal religions increasing memberships in Central America. Crosses, rosary beads, or figures of saints may be important. Female children may be protected from "evil eye" (*mal ojo*) by red earrings because red is "strong" color offering protection. Male babies may wear red knitted caps; both sexes may wear red *bolsita*—little bag of herbs placed around neck to protect from harm. Check with parents before removing any red item on baby.

* **Self-care.** General expectation that they will be cared for when in hospital. If nurse expects client to participate in care, specific instructions necessary.

Food Practices
* **Usual meal pattern.** Three meals daily, lunch the major meal, perhaps followed by traditional siesta or nap. Evening meal usually smaller and served later in evening. Rice common. Traditional foods spicy. In traditional Mayan culture, man sits down to eat and wife serves him, eating separately from husband.
* **Food beliefs and rituals.** Many Central Americans believe psychophysical state or condition to be related to strong-weak or hot-cold influences. An ill person is said to be too hot, too cold, chilled, or weakened by a variety of causes. Qualities of hot and cold also ascribed to foods and liquids, but have no relationship to actual temperature. If person has "hot" illness, "cold" foods used to restore balance. Some Central Americans may believe if time for meal has passed without eating, one's appetite diminishes, and best to wait until next meal rather than eating in between meals. No ice in drinks. Serve liquids at room temperature.
* **Usual diet.** Coffee and tortillas or bread common for breakfast. Soups, meat, rice (or beans), and vegetables for main meal at noon. Tamales a traditional food enjoyed by many.
* **Fluids.** Fluids generally served at room temperature. Many enjoy very sweet coffee.
* **Food prohibitions.** Avoid drinking or eating "cold" food while participating in "hot" activities such as ironing. Some persons believe cold food (ice cream) or iced beverages cause stomach pain. Raw fruits and vegetables often avoided because thought to cause illnesses. Certain foods (milk, avocados) might be avoided by women during menses.
* **Food prescriptions.** Tortillas and beans are staples. Be punctual with meals.

Symptom Management
* **Pain.** Offer pain medication as ordered. Pain viewed as necessary part of life to be endured. May be viewed as consequence of "earthly misconduct or "imbalance" of nature. Expression

pain (moaning or crying) acceptable.

* **Dyspnea.** Anxious when dyspneic. Use of oxygen or other "high tech" interventions viewed as sign of increasing gravity of illness.

* **Nausea/vomiting.** Vomiting uncomfortable and embarrassing in presence of others. Over-the-counter medications such as Alka Seltzer may be taken. At home, clients may take laxative to "purge" stomach.

* **Constipation/diarrhea.** May be attributed to eating spoiled or bad food. Men may be reluctant to disclose symptoms to female RN. Will accept enemas with reluctance and embarrassment.

* **Fatigue.** Attributed to lack of vitamins and proper food or may be associated with preoccupation or worry. Men may be reluctant to report fatigue because maleness associated with strength. Central Americans from *campesino* (peasant) backgrounds associate fatigue with overwork rather than illness.

* **Depression.** Attributed to tangible event (such as death of a family member) or an illness. Associated with family problems or being away from family. Sometimes somatized. Those who have experienced catastrophic life events associated with political violence or war may suffer posttraumatic stress syndrome.

* **Self-care for symptom management.** Over-the-counter medications frequently used. Because many Central Americans very poor, may fail to seek early or preventive care.

Birth Rituals/Care of the New Mother/Baby

* **Pregnancy care.** Latin culture values mothers and babies. Pregnant woman given much attention, encouraged to eat well and rest often. Culturally specific beliefs about avoiding cool air, not eating "hot" foods. Strong emotional states to be avoided. Some believe that strong moonlight will cause birth defect in baby.

* **Labor practices.** May vocalize expression of pain and discomfort. Often pregnant woman's mother wants to be with her during delivery. Customary for several women to attend to mother.

* **Role of the laboring woman during birth process.** Mother usually active in delivery. Other women present offer

encouragement and advice. Mother may scream and become emotional.

* **Role of the father and other family members during birth process.** Fathers usually have passive role. Father may wish to be with his wife; in Mayan culture, father expected to be there to "see how mother suffers."

* **Vaginal vs. cesarean section.** Vaginal delivery preferred. Cesarean section viewed as serious event, possibly detrimental to health of mother.

* **Breastfeeding.** Varies by social class. Mothers of higher income may prefer to bottle feed. Working mothers may breastfeed concurrently with bottle feeding or may choose bottle feeding entirely. Breastfeeding occurs in public. "Strong" foods, such as avocados, may be avoided.

* **Birth recuperation.** Some mothers may follow practice of *La Cuarenta*—specified period of time after delivery with dietary and rest prescriptions. New mothers must avoid "cold" foods or drinks as well as drafts of cold air. Mother believed to be in "cold" state and should eat or drink "hot" substances and keep herself physically warm. "Cold" foods or drinks will also make mother's milk "cold," causing infant to become ill. New mothers should avoid strong emotional states. After childbirth, woman considered in "weak" state, needing to exert special precautions during postnatal period. Certain foods (such as chicken soup, bananas, and meat) thought to "strengthen" mother. Herbal teas and baths may be used for mother and baby.

* **Problems with baby.** Talk to mother with father present (e.g., "I'm worried that..." and "I think you should..."). Aunts and grandmothers provide advice for infant care. Prescriptions followed regarding "hot" and "cold" qualities. Babies often dressed "too warmly" by U.S. standards.

* **Male and female circumcision.** Traditionally, male circumcision not done at birth. However, if parents wish to adhere to U.S. patterns of behavior and infant care, may provide consent for male circumcision. Female circumcision never done.

Death Rituals

* **Preparation.** Eldest male of family should be informed of impending death. Catholic clients and families may want priest to administer sacrament.
* **Home vs. hospital.** If possible, most Central Americans would prefer to die with dignity at home, surrounded by family members.
* **Special needs.** Nurse can assure an atmosphere of privacy and quiet for sacrament of the sick. If patient can swallow, glass of water can be provided to help patient swallow small wafer-like host. Candles may be used if patient not receiving oxygen.
* **Care of the body.** Traditionally, family members prepare the body for burial. Nurse should ask if they wish to prepare the body for mortuary. Death considered spiritual event, and family members will want to say goodbye to deceased person.
* **Attitudes toward organ donation.** Acceptable if body treated with respect. Cremation not common practice.
* **Attitudes toward autopsy.** Body should be treated with respect. All family members may be involved in decision. Mayan families may not be comfortable with autopsy.

Family Relationships

* **Composition/structure.** Extended families common; relationships among members close. Gay and lesbian family members are not acknowledged.
* **Decision making.** Father or eldest son primary decision maker.
* **Spokesperson.** Father or eldest son.
* **Gender issues.** Both men and women have traditionally defined roles. Women's roles confined to home and family.
* **Caring role.** Women care for sick. Sometimes men fulfill aspects of this role; may be very caring and attentive to sick mother.
* **Expectations of and for children.** Children may be "pampered" by U.S. standards. Discipline may be more casual. Education valued more for men than women.
* **Expectations of and for elders.** Great respect for elders in all Central American societies. Families expected to care for elders.

* **Expectations of adults in caring for children and elders.** Most Central American families reluctant to place elder family member in nursing home.
* **Expectation of visitors.** Central Americans very family oriented, and many may visit patient in hospital. Orient to unit and encourage family to participate in care.

Spiritual/Religious Orientation

* **Primary religious/spiritual affiliation.** Traditionally, Central Americans are Catholic although many have been converted to Pentecostal religions. Mayan Indians may adhere to beliefs associated with combination of 16th century Catholicism and Mayan mythology.
* **Usual religious/spiritual practices.** Catholics recite rosary and use services of priest for confession, communion, or sacrament of sick. Members of Pentecostal churches may attend revivals, prayer meetings, and actively proselytize.
* **Use of spiritual healing/healers.** Priest or physician may be summoned. Advice of traditional healers known as *curanderos(as)* may be sought.

Illness Beliefs

* **Causes of physical illness.** Ill health a result of imbalance; thus, concern with hot, cold, strong, and weak. Physical illnesses also caused or aggravated by strong emotions, such as anger, fright, and sadness. Illness also attributed to outside sources such as evil eye (*mal ojo*), witch's curse, or ghost. "Bad wind" or "forces" may enter body directly and cause illness.
* **Causes of mental illness.** Abnormal behavior, especially depression, may be attributed to significant life event such as death of husband, birth of child, etc. Intense or strong emotions, such as anger, grief, surprise may lead to sadness, anxiety, or nervousness. Nervios or "nerves" a common state of anxiety or worry. Mental illnesses may be attributed to supernatural.
* **Causes of genetic defects.** May be attributed to mother's behavior during pregnancy (strenuous activities, not resting or eating properly, failing to avoid

moonlight, especially during an eclipse). May be seen as God's will.

* **Sick role.** Sick person often assumes passive role, and family members provide care. Patient urged to eat nutritious food, avoid cold air, and get adequate rest for recovery.

* **Home and folk remedies.** Herbal teas common. Lemons, eggs, and "pure" water believed to have special healing and protective powers. Great reliance on over-the-counter medications.

* **Acceptance of procedures.** Procedures should be explained clearly. Some Central Americans may be reluctant to donate blood, believing it would make them "weak."

* **Care seeking.** Central Americans seek care from physicians, although this may be delayed because of cost. Most would prefer to see health professionals who speak Spanish, especially physicians. Many will also seek care from traditional healers such as curanderos if available. Many Central Americans will also visit pharmacies to inquire about appropriate medications.

Health Practices

* **Concept of health.** Good health related to balance of hot and cold, strong and weak. By nature, men considered stronger than women. Good health associated with ability to perform functional roles.

* **Health promotion and prevention.** Fresh air, eating well, resting, and enough sleep. Think positive thoughts, do not get angry, upset or hassled. Lemons and pure water have health promotive qualities. Laxatives for children will "keep them cleaned out."

* **Screening.** Respect for medical authority, and screening for various procedures should not be problem. Medical diagnosis readily disclosed to family.

Selected References

Andrews, M. M., & Boyle, J. S. (Eds.). (1995). *Transcultural concepts in nursing care* (2nd ed.). Philadelphia, PA: J. B. Lippincott Company.

Glittenberg, J. (1994). *To the mountain and back: The mysteries of Guatemalan highland family life.* Prospect Heights, IL: Waveland Press.

Villarruel, A. M., & Ortiz de Montellano, B. (1992). Culture and pain: A Mesoamerican perspective. *Advances in Nursing Science, 15,* 21-32.

Author

Joyceen S. Boyle, RN, PhD, FAAN is Professor and Chair of the Department of Community Nursing, Medical College of Georgia, Augusta, GA. Her teaching and research endeavors focus on women's health and qualitative research methods. Her dissertation research was conducted in Guatemala in 1979-1981.

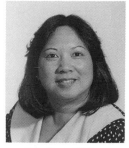

Pauline Chin

Cultural/Ethnic Identity
* **Preferred terms.** Chinese, Chinese American
* **History of immigration/migration.**

1840–1882	Chinese laborers came to U.S. for jobs; many employed to work on railroads.
1882	Chinese Exclusion Act - suspended immigration of Chinese to America.
1924	National Origins Quota Act - annual quota = 105 Chinese.
1965	National Origins Quota Act abolished. By 1970, U.S. Chinese population increased by 84 percent.

Chinese health practices vary according to length of time in U.S. Three major groups and health practices are:

Early immigrants—immigrated 40-60 years' ago, strongest believers in Chinese folk medicine.

Newer immigrants—immigrated in the past 20 years, combine both Chinese Folk and Western Medicine practices.

First and second generation Chinese Americans—mostly oriented to Western Medicine.

* **Map page.** *See Appendix C, p. 1.*

Communication
* **Major language(s) and dialects.** Cantonese and Mandarin most common.
* **Literacy assessment.** Ability to speak or read varies with individuals. Elderly Chinese (especially women) may be unable to read or write. Ask questions to ascertain understanding, but not questions that require only yes or no answer.
* **Nonverbal communication.** Eye contact and touching more common among family members and close friends; eye contact avoided with authority figures as sign

of respect. Keeping respectful distance recommended. Asking questions seen as disrespectful; silence may be sign of respect.

*   **Use of interpreters.** Family members usually available for interpreting needs, but professional interpreters recommended for translation about complicated medical procedures. Avoid male interpreters for older female patients due to modesty issues.

*   **Greetings.** Chinese people are often shy, especially in unfamiliar environment; socializing and friendly greetings helpful. Address older patients by Mr./Mrs. and last name. Use of first name could be viewed as disrespectful among older individuals.

*   **Tone of voice.** Chinese language is very expressive and often appears loud to non-Chinese people. Often this "loudness" is carried through to the English language and may appear unintentionally abrupt.

*   **Orientation toward time.** Being on time not valued by traditional Chinese societies. Reinforce importance of being on time for medical appointments.

*   **Consents.** Involve oldest male of the family with consent explanations, especially with young females. Out of respect, Chinese patients may not ask questions, but may nod politely at everything being said. Assess understanding by asking clear questions.

*   **Privacy.** Privacy very important; Chinese people usually extremely modest. To "save face," Chinese people may not want to disclose personal information to health providers. Involve close family members when necessary.

*   **Serious or terminal illness.** Some families may prefer to be present when addressing information concerning serious or terminal illness. Ensure involvement of head of household (usually eldest male member of the family).

Activities of Daily Living

*   **Modesty.** Chinese people are extremely modest, especially women. Avoid assigning male nurses to female patients.

*   **Skin care.** Good hygiene important. No special needs. Allow family to assist with bathing.

*   **Hair care.** Patients may not want to wash hair while sick.

* **Nail care.** No special needs.
* **Toileting.** Privacy important; using toilet preferred to use of bedpan or urinal.
* **Special clothing or amulets.** Good luck articles (jade, rope around waist) may be worn to ensure good health and good luck. Avoid removing articles; if removal is required, encourage family members to take articles/jewelry home for safety.
* **Self-care.** Most Chinese patients prefer to perform their own activities of daily living, but some older men may expect to be cared for by family members or staff.

Food Practices
* **Usual meal pattern.** Usually eat three meals a day, largest at dinner.
* **Special utensils.** Chopsticks, if available.
* **Food beliefs and rituals.** Food viewed as important in maintaining balance of Yin (cold) and Yang (hot) in the body. Imbalance of Yin and Yang believed to cause illness. Food also used to treat illness and disease. Patients may refuse certain foods due to beliefs about illness and which foods should be used to treat it. Obtain dietary consult when appropriate to determine food preferences and diet restrictions. Encourage families to bring in food from home if possible.
* **Usual diet.** Rice and noodles important staples in Chinese diet. Meat usually not eaten in large quantities and patients may prefer beef cooked until well done. Vegetables frequently eaten mixed with meat to maintain the balance of Yin and Yang. Chinese prefer vegetables cooked, not raw.
* **Fluids.** Chinese people drink plenty of hot liquids, especially tea, when sick. Hot beverages preferred due to belief that cold water shocks the system.
* **Food prohibitions.** Food considered Yin (cold) or Yang (hot) depending on the Yin or Yang energy it is thought to yield when metabolized. Yin foods include: fruits, vegetables, cold liquids, and beer. Yang foods include: meats, eggs, hot soup and liquids, oily and fried foods. Illness caused by Yang excesses are treated with Yin foods, and Yang foods are avoided, and vice versa.
* **Food prescriptions.** Based on information above, family members may bring in special foods to help treat illnesses.

Consult with Dietary to ensure compliance with diet. Some Chinese also use herbal preparations and special soups to treat illnesses. Sometimes difficult to determine content of these special preparations.

Symptom Management

* **Pain.** Patient may not complain of pain; be aware of non-verbal cues to assess pain. Offer pain medications instead of waiting for patient to ask for them. Some patients may use acupressure or acupuncture to treat pain or illness.
* **Dyspnea.** Caused by too much *Yin*. Some patients will treat with hot soups/ broths and wear warm clothes.
* **Nausea/vomiting.** Caused by too much *Yin*. Will treat with hot soups/broths.
* **Constipation/diarrhea.** Caused by too much *Yang*. Some patients will treat with fruits, vegetables, and other *Yin* foods.
* **Fatigue.** Caused by too much *Yin*. Will treat with hot soups/broths. *Ginseng* a common remedy.
* **Depression.** Mental health problems and depression viewed as shameful and not readily discussed.
* **Self-care for symptom management.** Most Chinese treat minor symptoms with food remedies as discussed earlier. However, many major illnesses (i.e., cancer, heart disease) ignored until advanced; some patients will seek Western medicine for treatment.

Birth Rituals/Care of the New Mother/Baby

* **Pregnancy care.** Believe that certain activities will affect baby during pregnancy (i.e., going to the zoo during pregnancy will cause baby to look like one of animals). Pregnancy considered a "cold" condition and *Yin* foods should be avoided (i.e., eating watermelon during pregnancy will cause the baby to have asthma).
* **Labor practices.** No special practices.
* **Role of the laboring woman during birth process.** Although Chinese are stoic in nature, it is acceptable for Chinese women to exhibit pain by moaning, etc., during childbirth.
* **Role of the father and other family members during birth process.** Usually female family members present during birth process. Father and other male

members do not normally play active role.

* **Vaginal vs. cesarean section.** Vaginal delivery preferred.
* **Breastfeeding.** Breastfeeding usually preferred over bottle feeding unless mother works. While breastfeeding, mother is expected to ingest *Yang* ("hot") foods to strengthen health of baby.
* **Birth recuperation.** During first 30 days post-partum, mother's pores believed to remain open and cold air can enter the body. Based on this belief, new Chinese mother may be forbidden to go outdoors or take a shower or bath. Diet will be high in *Yang* foods (i.e., meat, eggs, liver) and *Yin* foods may be avoided. Many mothers will ingest specially prepared soups and broths containing pigs' feet and chicken.
* **Problems with baby.** New baby is center of focus and attention in Chinese family. Problems with baby should be addressed with head of household and treated with utmost importance.
* **Male and female circumcision.** Although female circumcision not performed, male circumcision quite common.

Death Rituals

* **Preparation.** Chinese patients may be fatalistic when faced with terminal illness and death and may not want to talk about it. Family may prefer that patient not be told about terminal illness, or may prefer to tell patient themselves.
* **Home vs. hospital.** Many believe that people go to hospitals to die because dying at home will bring bad luck. Others believe that the spirit might get lost if death occurs in hospital.
* **Special needs.** Special amulets and cloths may be brought from home to be placed on the body.
* **Care of the body.** Some families prefer to bathe their family member after death.
* **Attitudes toward organ donation.** Believe that body should be kept intact. Organ donation not common.
* **Attitudes toward autopsy.** Body should be kept intact so autopsies may not be allowed.

Family Relationships

* **Composition/structure.** Extended families common. Two or three generations often live in same household. Wife

expected to become part of husband's family. Gay and lesbian relationships are not acknowledged—considered shameful for family.

* **Decision making.** Patriarchal society. Oldest male makes decisions.
* **Spokesperson.** Usually oldest male in household.
* **Gender issues.** Males usually more highly respected and valued than females.
* **Caring role.** Caring role usually responsibility of a female in household (mother, wife, daughter, daughter-in-law).
* **Expectations of and for children.** Children highly valued in Chinese families, expected to respect their elders. Education highly valued. Children who do not do well in school bring shame to family.
* **Expectations of and for elders.** Elders very respected and honored. In extended care families, grandparents often responsible for care of grandchildren.
* **Expectations of adults in caring for children and elders.** Families expected to care for children and elders, rather than leave them in day care or institutions. Mothers often expected to stay at home to raise their children if another family member is not available to babysit.
* **Expectation of visitors.** Common for great numbers of family members/friends to visit Chinese patient. Considered polite for visitors to bring food or gifts

Spiritual/Religious Orientation

* **Primary religious/spiritual affiliation.** Many Chinese are Buddhists. Catholic and Protestant religions also common.
* **Usual religious/spiritual practices.** Common for Chinese families to honor their ancestors, especially during major holidays such as Chinese New Year. Incense burning and eating special foods usually occurs during special occasions. Good luck symbols may be displayed in homes.
* **Use of spiritual healing/healers.** Some Chinese use herbalists and acupuncturists in conjunction with Western medicine or before seeking medical help. Rarely, healer will be sought to rid psychiatric patients of evil spirits.

Illness Beliefs

*   **Causes of physical illness.** Most physical illnesses caused by imbalance of *Yin* and *Yang* in the body.
*   **Causes of mental illness.** Mental illness thought to be caused by a lack of harmony of emotions. In some cases, thought to be caused by evil spirits. Mental wellness occurs when psychologic and physiologic functions are integrated.
*   **Causes of genetic defects.** Genetic defects usually blamed on the mother, generally something she did or ate.
*   **Sick role.** Sick role common in the Chinese patient. Family expected to take care of patient, and patient takes passive role in his/her illness.
*   **Home and folk remedies.** *Ginseng* root a commonly used home remedy for a number of ailments including: anemia, colic, depression, indigestion, impotence, and rheumatism. Other Chinese remedies include: deer antlers for strengthening bones and treating impotence, turtle shells to stimulate weak kidneys and to remove gallstones, and snake flesh for healthy eyes and clear vision.
*   **Acceptance of procedures.** Some Chinese are fearful of having blood drawn, believing that it will weaken the body. Many Chinese avoid surgery due to belief that body needs to be kept intact so soul will have a place to live when making future visits to earth.
*   **Care seeking.** Many Chinese use home remedies for minor ailments such as colds and skin diseases. Most Chinese seek Western doctors for more serious ailments such as cancer. In making a decision for seeking care, advice of relatives and friends will be sought. Professional Chinese practitioners prescribe herbs and acupuncture based on diagnosis involving *Yin/Yang* and energy balance.

Health Practices

*   **Concept of health.** Health is maintaining balance between *Yin* and *Yang* influences, not only in the body but in the environment. Harmony important to maintain with body, mind, and spirit.
*   **Health promotion and prevention.** Preventing illness and promoting good health means that one should eat a

diet balanced with *Yin* and *Yang* foods. Also important to maintain harmony with family and friends.

* **Screening.** When screening Chinese patients, be aware of Chinese beliefs and health practices. Allow family involvement and participation, and respect privacy issues. For communication barriers, interpreters recommended.

Selected References

Chung, H.J. (1977). Understanding the oriental maternity patient. *Nursing Clinics of North America, 12*(1), 67-75.

Harwood, A. (Ed.) (1981). *Ethnicity and medical care* (pp. 131-171). Cambridge, MA: Harvard University Press.

Lin, Tsung-Yi. (1983). Psychiatry and Chinese culture. *The Western Journal of Medicine, 139*(6), 862-867.

Mo, B. (1992). Modesty, sexuality, and breast health in Chinese-American women. *The Western Journal of Medicine, 157*(3), 260-264.

Rawl, S.M. (1992). Perspectives on nursing care of Chinese Americans. *Journal of Holistic Nursing, 10*(1), 6-17.

Author
Pauline Chin, RN, MS is a Nurse Manager at the Medical Center at University of California, San Francisco. She is a second generation Chinese American who has done numerous presentations on health care practices and beliefs of Chinese patients.

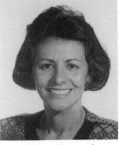

*Pilar Bernal
de Pheils*

Cultural/Ethnic Identity

* **Preferred terms.** Colombians (English) *Colombianos* (Spanish)
* **History of immigration.** Colombians have been coming to U.S. since 1950s more or less steadily, mainly for economic reasons. Some also have come in past ten years for political reasons.
* **Map page.** *See Appendix C, p. 2.*

Communication

* **Major language(s) and dialects.** Spanish is national language. Natives of San Andres and Providencia Islands speak dialect *Papiamento*, mixture of English, French, and Spanish.
* **Literacy assessment.** Literacy level may vary based upon socioeconomic background. Colombians of high socioeconomic background may speak, read, and write English well, particularly young to middle-aged adults.
* **Nonverbal communication.** Typically very affectionate and friendly. Appropriate to touch when confronted with hardship (i.e., giving bad news). Health professional may hold patient's hand or put a hand on patient's shoulder. Colombians may not have direct eye contact in presence of authority figure (MD, RN) or in awkward situation. Respectful of elders and authority figures. Silence may mean failure to understand what has been said and embarrassment about asking or disagreeing. Personal space close and frequently shared with family members or close friends.
* **Use of interpreters.** May use family members as interpreters. May need professional interpreter if family member not an adult. When sensitive issues (sexual history) need to be discussed, choose

close family member of same gender if possible.

* **Greetings.** As sign of respect, address middle aged and elderly as Mrs. (*Señora*), Mr. (*Señor*), or Miss (*Señorita*) followed by their last name. If woman is single, carefully address her as Miss. If using Spanish use the word *Usted* for second person ("you"). Men shake hands with men and women. Instead of shaking hands with each other, women clasp each other's wrists. Greetings between friends or relatives are hand to hand between men, or cheek to cheek between women and also between women and men.

* **Tone of voice.** Raised tone of voice in presence of family members or friends. May get agitated or emotional when nervous or frightened. Important to request politely and avoid using loud voice when talking to them.

* **Orientation toward time.** Colombians unaccustomed to long term planning; most plans are for short term. May be few minutes late for appointments. Need to emphasize importance of keeping appointments, cancelling if necessary with some warning. Social gathering time always expected to start later than announced time.

* **Consents.** Written consent forms not customary in Colombia. Need to begin consent process by explaining that most procedures in this country require written and signed form from patient. Explain slowly, obtain frequent feedback from patient, and allow questions. Patient may be embarrassed to ask questions.

* **Privacy.** Sensitive to concept of shame (*verguenza*). Strong respect for authority will allow disclosure of private information if relevant to care. Include family members when necessary, particularly if patient requests their presence.

* **Serious or terminal illness.** Consult with close family member on how to communicate news; family may choose to disclose news to patient or may ask you do it, or to be present at this time. Family members may choose not to disclose seriousness of illness to patient, particularly in case of chi' sick elderly parent.

Activities of Daily Living

*   **Modesty.** Very modest, particularly if patient is opposite gender to provider. Offer gown and robe to patient.
*   **Skin care.** Customary to shower daily. Patient may choose not to shower if feeling weak/feverish or if medically contraindicated. Most women shave their legs and axillae daily; men also shave their faces daily.
*   **Hair care.** Customarily hair not washed daily.
*   **Nail care.** Women prefer long nails and use nail file instead of scissors. Men cut their nails very short with scissors and, if not very sick, may prefer to do it themselves.
*   **Toileting.** If there is need to use bedpan or urinal, protect privacy.
*   **Special clothing/amulets.** Predominantly Roman Catholic. If possible, allow use of medallions (*escapularios*), rosary beads, religious figures/pictures.
*   **Self-care.** Hospitalized patient expects to be taken care of regarding most of usual self-care activities. At home most self-care activities expected to be done by close family member.

Food Practices

*   **Usual meal pattern.** Three meals a day. Lunch larger than dinner.
*   **Food beliefs and rituals.** Food served at every social occasion. Diet varies by region. Rural people hold more strongly to traditional diets than those from urban areas. Food beliefs influenced by Catholicism (e.g., Lent, Holy Week).
*   **Usual diet.** Coffee and bread part of breakfast; rice and potatoes a staple at lunch and for some also at dinner. Soup common for lunch. Fruit juice always accompanies meals. Vegetables scarce in their diet (common salad has only tomato, lettuce and carrot). May snack between meals. Sandwiches do not replace meals.
*   **Fluids.** Prefer to drink fruit juices diluted with water.
*   **Food prohibitions.** Most Catholics eat fish on Fridays during Lent. Prefer hot/warm drinks first thing in the morning. Women avoid acidic food during menstruation.
*   **Food prescriptions.** Warm/bland fluids/foods

when sick. Meat broth instead of chicken soup when sick. *Agua de panela* (a drink of unprocessed sugar and water), frequently used when sick, particularly for respiratory/flu symptoms.

Symptom Management

* **Pain.** (*Dolor*) Occasionally, patient may report feeling *inflamada(o)* indicating abdominal pain. Women may be more expressive than men when in pain, tend to cry easily. Use pain medications as directed, prefer oral or IV routes over IM or rectal. Fearful of becoming addicted to pain medications. Heat/ice used to control pain.
* **Dyspnea.** To be without air or unable to breathe. *Quedarse sin aire* or *no poder respirar* are common expressions of dyspnea. Patient/relatives may be very anxious when this happens. Oxygen accepted and expected when this occurs.
* **Nausea/vomiting.** (*Nausea/vomito*) Will feel embarrassed after vomiting. Will accept medications offered to control symptoms.
* **Constipation/diarrhea.** (*Estrenimiento* or *estar dura del estomago*-constipation) Bowel movement expected daily and will be a concern if none occurs. Will accept enemas if necessary. Loose stools in any form reported as diarrhea. Milk usually stopped if diarrhea occurs.
* **Fatigue.** (*Cansada*) Will accept medications but may be fearful of addiction if sleeping pills necessary. Naps taken to relieve fatigue.
* **Depression.** Depressed people say "I am sad" (*Triste*). Depression not talked about openly.
* **Self-care for symptom management.** Not expected; may not take action until very sick.

Birth Rituals/Care of the New Mother/Baby

* **Pregnancy care.** Expected if patient/family ca afford. If immigrant from rural areas, may not be expected regardless of eco nomics. Pregnant women protected from hard labor and encouraged by family members to rest and eat wel
* **Labor practices.** Laboring women do not during labor for fear of vomiting; only sips of fluid. Most prefer to

down while in labor, but may walk and/or shower early in labor. Relatives generally not present during labor and delivery but will welcome the option in U.S. Analgesia welcome but not expected in lower socioeconomic groups since not offered routinely to poor women in Colombian hospitals.

* **Role of the laboring woman during birth process.** Passive, may vary in expression of pain, from being very noisy to suffering in silence.

* **Role of the father and other family members during birth process.** Family members not expected to be present at delivery, but younger fathers may welcome the opportunity. If present, mother of laboring woman plays major role in supporting daughter.

* **Vaginal vs. cesarean section.** Cesarean section may be sign of upper class status and requested when in much pain.

* **Breastfeeding.** Expected, particularly in low to middle socioeconomic groups. Although breastfeeding has increased at all socio-economic levels, length of time varies from weeks/months (if woman has to work outside home) up to a year. Few will continue beyond a year; however, longer period expected if from rural area.

* **Birth recuperation.** Mothers and babies cared for by female relatives, specifically mothers and sisters. Not allowed to do strenuous physical activities and, in some cases, particularly if from rural areas, do not leave house until passage of 40 days of *dieta* (postpartum). Some postpartum women may cover their ears with cotton to avoid "air entering their system." Father may play participatory role in care of new mother and baby. Mother's diet rich in protein; lots of chicken for first month. Most women shower on second day postpartum and peri-care may be done by female relative.

* **Problems with baby.** If problem with baby, first approach father or, in his absence, close relative (her mother, if present) to suggest best way to present information to mother. Authority figure such as MD should transmit information.

Male and female circumcision. Female circumcision never performed. Male circumcision varies, traditionally done at

birth if parents prefer. Decision not
influenced by religion.

Death Rituals

* **Preparation.** Inform head of family (parents or
   eldest child), preferably away from
   patient's room. Offer services of
   Catholic priest for patient to receive
   sacrament. Difficult decisions often
   discussed among close family members.

* **Home vs. hospital.** If illness acute, may
   choose hospital. If disease terminal
   after chronic illness, may prefer to
   die at home.

* **Special needs.** May be surrounded by all family
   members except small children.
   Catholic prayer commonly used at
   patient's bedside. Patient may ask for
   priest. Family members may cry
   uncontrollably and loudly; women
   may be hysterical.

* **Care of the body.** All family members may
   want to see body before it is taken to
   morgue. Other than cleaning and
   dressing, no special preparation of
   body customarily done by family.
   Minimal preparation of body done otherwise, since at home Colombians generally buried within 24 to 36 hours of
   death. Cremation not common.
      A Colombian may need to be
   warned that in the U.S. the body
   is rarely buried before three days
   after death.

* **Attitudes toward organ donation.** May be
   acceptable to ask for organ donation.
   Ask closest family member, who may
   consult and decide with family. Present
   as act of goodness from family and as
   way to benefit other persons.

* **Attitudes toward autopsy.** Accepted if viewed
   as necessary to clarify cause of death.

Family Relationships

* **Composition/structure.** Nuclear family or
   single woman family. Family-oriented
   culture. Extended family very influential, if present, particularly if older
   generation. Being gay or lesbian not
   openly accepted. Patient/family will
   keep this information secret; close
   family members may be supportive.

* **Decision making.** Father or oldest sibling a
   as spokesperson; wife and other siblings part of decision making, par
   larly if siblings are adults.

* **Spokesperson.** Father or eldest sibling.

* **Gender issues.** Men make most decisions; women take caregiver role for any family member regardless of gender.
* **Caring role.** Women (mother, sister, or close relative) expected to take caring role. Patient pampered with attention and services to point of interfering with appropriate care such as beginning early ambulation and self-care activities (eating, bathing).
* **Expectations of and for children.** Highly protected and very dependent on parents. Children (adolescents) expected to live with parents until they marry unless study or work necessitates living elsewhere. Future plans of children heavily influenced by parental opinions. Parents emphasize punishment rather than positive rewards by frightening children. Mothers frequently threaten children with getting an injection if they're not well behaved in hospital or clinic. Taught to be quiet and avoid confrontations with parents and older persons, to be obedient, respectful, and shy.
* **Expectations of and for elders.** Treated with respect. They expect and are cared for by family members when ill. If economically dependent, they expect to live with one of children, usually daughter. Frequently babysit to allow their children and spouses to work.
* **Expectations of adults in caring for children and elders.** Adults, particularly adult women, expected to care for the sick. Institutionalization of family member a last resort, only in case of very sick family member with no adult family members able to stay home. Institutionalization regarded as abandonment of sick person. Boarding school for children may be acceptable if needed.
* **Expectation of visitors.** Expect many visits by relatives and friends when family member hospitalized. Accepted to ask respectfully to limit number of visitors. They may become noisy, particularly if patient not very ill.

Spiritual/Religious Orientation

* **Primary religious/spiritual affiliation.** Predominantly Catholic.
* **Usual religious/spiritual practices.** Religious family members (usually mother/grandmother) may recite prayers or rosary if

patient very ill. Call for priest to visit—whether for confession, communion, or receiving sacrament of the sick.

* **Use of spiritual healing/healers.** If patient extremely ill, presence of priest very important for purposes mentioned above. Nurses should facilitate priest-patient privacy.

Illness Beliefs

* **Causes of physical illness.** Severe illness may be attributed to God's design (purpose). Some may associate illness with bad behavior or punishment (i.e., if sick person has drinking problems, disease attributed to drinking).
* **Causes of mental illness.** May be explained as result of overwhelming situation. Believed that mental illness in women results from love deceptions. Mental illness stigmatizes family.
* **Causes of genetic defects.** Child with a genetic defect may be explained by parents, particularly mother, doing something wrong. Family members will accept loved ones with genetic defects and, if possible, prefer to care for them at home.
* **Sick role.** Sick person expects to be cared for during illness, usually by a female family member. Patient assumes passive role and lets family make decisions in relation to his/her care.
* **Home and folk remedies.** Herbal teas used very frequently before seeking medical care. Patients may self medicate with remedies from Colombia, since most medications can be bought there without prescription. Pharmacies in Colombia important, and, in many cases, primary source of health care. Always ask if patient is taking any medication given by friend or relative or sent from Colombia.
* **Acceptance of procedures.** Procedures well accepted if explained clearly and slowly. May accept need to donate blood, have surgery, or organ transplant if felt to be necessary.
* **Care seeking.** Western medicine expected and preferred in case of severe illness, but concurrent use of native healer (curandero[a]) may be present, particularly lower socioeconomic class.

Health Practices

* **Concept of health.** To be healthy is to be able to perform in expected role as mother/father, worker, others. Health associated with feeling good and happy.

* **Health promotion and prevention.** Interpreted as being and looking clean, and being able to rest and sleep well. Eating right very important for prevention of illness. Otherwise, people don't consciously do anything to promote their health, such as exercise. However, some educated people exercise for health promotion.

* **Screening.** Vaccination very important and adhered to for children. Women participate in more screening practices than men.

Selected References

Bernal, P., & Meleis, A. F. (1995). Self-care actions of Colombian por dia domestic workers: On prevention and care. *Women & Health, 22*(4), 77-95.

Author

Pilar Bernal de Pheils, RN, MS, FNP is Assistant Clinical Professor in the Family/Women's Primary Health Care Program, School of Nursing, University of California, San Francisco. She immigrated from Colombia in 1990 and since has worked as a faculty member and as an FNP in a community health clinic providing care to a large group of Latino women, including Colombians.

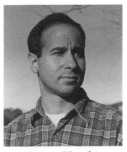

Larry Varela

Cultural/Ethnic Identity

* **Preferred terms.** Cuban may be used
    in referring to either native born or
    American born. Cubans very proud
    of their heritage, often do not see a
    need to identify themselves as
    American. Cuban American for
    American born.

* **History of immigration.**

    1895–1905   Influx to Tampa and Miami,
    Florida to assist with tobacco
    industry. Established small,
    tight communities.

    1940s–1950s Increased trade and commerce
    between U.S. and Cuba during
    WWII. Influx of workers for
    war industry.

    1959–1979   Largest immigration of Cubans
    due to overthrow of government
    and establishment of communist
    system by Fidel Castro. At this
    time, most middle and upper class-
    es left Cuba for U.S. Most immi-
    grants settled in Miami, Tampa,
    and New York and built strong
    communities. By living within
    these communities, were able to
    sustain much of their culture
    and language.

    1980   Mariel Boat Lift. 120,000 Cubans
    immigrated within the year. Many
    criminals were among this popula-
    tion as Castro emptied his jails.
    This population had lived with
    Communism for some 20 years
    and thus were socially different
    from previous immigrants.

    1981–present. Continued immigration of
    relatives of those already in U.S.
    Economic conditions in Cuba cur-
    rently stimulating more emigrants.

* **Map page.** *See Appendix C, p. 2.*

Communication

* **Major language(s) and dialects.** Castilian
Spanish (Common Spanish). Cubans
speak Spanish quickly and shorten
words by dropping letters. Also have
incorporated many English words into
spoken Spanish which are not used by
other Spanish speakers, for example,
lonchar, taken from English for lunch.
In Castilian Spanish, the word for
lunch is *almorzar*.
* **Literacy assessment.** Cubans have a high
degree of literacy. Cubans who arrived
in America at a young age and those
American born are often fluent in
both English and Spanish. Older
Cubans living in U.S. for many years
vary in their command of English,
depending on their assimilation, need,
and location of residency. New arrivals
often speak little or no English.
* **Nonverbal communication.** Cubans typically
outgoing and confronting. Close contact and touching acceptable and sign
of affection among family and friends.
Direct eye contact expected during
conversation. Looking away shows lack
of respect or dishonesty. Silence usually means awkwardness or uncertainty.
Cubans often use hand gestures to add
emphasis or drama when talking.
* **Use of interpreters.** Prefer most educated or
acculturated family member. Discuss
sensitive topics such as terminal prognosis or sex related issues only with
older immediate family members.
Discuss HIV/AIDS diagnosis only with
patient. Another health provider
should translate when HIV/AIDS
diagnosis given.
* **Greetings.** Only formal at first introduction.
After that, familiar tone and address
used. Handshake common among men.
Elderly people shown more respect.
Family members and close friends greet
by embracing and kissing on cheek.
* **Tone of voice.** Cubans speak loudly in normal
conversation. Commands or requests
are direct and often forceful. To an
outsider, conversation may seem hos-
tile and aggressive.
* **Orientation toward time.** Cubans often
follow Western business time.
Orientation to social time varies
greatly. Emphasis often on future
but strongly influenced by

socioeconomic status. Elderly Cubans
or newer arrivals may focus more on
past and possible return to Cuba.

* **Consents.** Use interpreter when needed. Often
family will wish to consult with most
educated, respected, or eldest family
member before giving consent.
Knowledge of hazards or possible side
effects usually not desired and withheld from patient because thought to
cause unwanted stress or actual occurrence of problem. Cubans usually do
not like to be involved in research for
fear of not obtaining best treatment for
themselves. Most are comfortable in
signing written consent.

* **Privacy.** Extremely important to Cubans. Only
family members appointed by patient
or person directing care should be
included in discussions. Sensitive or
personal information may be withheld
from health care workers due to social
implications. Often family will prefer
information to be withheld from
patients themselves. Discuss this issue
with family before informing patient.
Often this withholding of information
is requested by patient.

* **Serious or terminal illness.** Acculturated
Cubans will want to be informed of
their terminal illness. Less acculturated
will probably follow cultural norms:
first informing spouse, eldest child or
person directing care, then immediate
family will be included as appropriate.
Allow family to inform patient. Often
they will not disclose this information
to patient, believing that knowledge
would affect his or her will to live
and thus minimize fight for life.
Pregnant women, children, and ill
family members often excluded from
such discussion or knowledge.

Do not resuscitate (DNR) orders
usually not acceptable to Cubans. Feel
strongly that everything possible
should be done for patient. Agreeing
to DNR shows giving up hope and
allowing patient to die, seen by others
as uncaring and abandonment. Could
also be interpreted as assisting with or
hoping for death. Fear of death quite
strong among Cubans.

Activities of Daily Living
* **Modesty.** Very modest—both men and women.
Provide adequate covering. Women

patients prefer female nurses but will accept males.

* **Skin care.** Daily washing preferred.
* **Hair care.** Normally shampoo daily but during illness less frequently. Believe that wet hair may cause chills/draft and exacerbate illness. Some women will not wash hair during menses.
* **Nail care.** Nail care important to women even during illness. Women usually wear nails long.
* **Toileting.** Regularity is priority for many. Prefer not to use bedpans because of uncleanliness, awkwardness, and lack of privacy. Will argue to use bathroom for privacy, cleanliness, and to conduct good peri-care, often with soap and water.
* **Special clothing/amulets.** Will pin religious medallions, rosary beads, or cross to bed or clothing. Take care when discarding sheets or gown.
* **Self-care.** Patient's role is well defined as totally submissive in all care activities. Female family members will conduct all activities if allowed, including bathing, toileting, and feeding in hospital or at home. Concept of self-care as part of recovery not accepted.

Food Practices

* **Usual meal pattern.** Three meals a day. Elderly or new arrivals still make lunch main meal.
* **Food beliefs and rituals.** During illness important to eat fresh foods, soups, and broths. Often believe that not good to eat too much when ill. Some foods may be omitted during illness because too difficult to digest (type may vary).
* **Usual diet.** Rice and beans common with lunch and dinner. Most foods fried. Meat important with all meals. Small variety of vegetables eaten. Sweets eaten frequently.
* **Fluids.** Cold fluids, juices, and coffee.
* **Food prohibitions.** Forbidden to drink water when eating fish or to drink beer when eating bananas.
* **Food prescriptions.** Many used as home remedies.

Symptom Management

* **Pain.** (*Dolor*) Culturally acceptable to express feeling of pain. Men may seem hypersensitive. Women more tolerant. Understand numerical scale of

expressing pain. Fear becoming addicted to narcotics. Prefer not to take medication or to wean off as quickly as possible. Injections viewed as more effective or stronger than tablets. Non-pharmacological methods for pain control usually under-utilized.

* **Dyspnea.** (*Corto de aire* - Short of breath) May become very expressive during dyspnea. Understands numerical scale. Easy acceptance of oxygen. Non-pharmacological methods for controlling dyspnea useful.

* **Nausea/vomiting.** (*Nausea/Vomito*) Often explained as nervous stomach due to stress or nervousness. Viewed as marker for increasing illness. Will quickly report vomiting. Rectal administration of medication easily accepted.

* **Constipation/diarrhea.** (*Estrenimiento/Diarrea*) Constipation could mean poor eating habits. Diarrhea could be caused by eating something which did not agree with you, or by anxiety, or illness. Lengthy discussion around bowels not uncommon. Accepting of medical treatments such as enemas, suppositories, or nutritional controls.

* **Fatigue.** (*Fatiga*) Cubans do not customarily take naps in the afternoon. Will report fatigue. Understand numerical scale of expressing fatigue. Probably more accepting of non-pharmacological than medical treatments.

* **Depression.** (*Depresion*) Often ignored or denied. May be attributed to "nerves," extreme stress, or anxiety. Viewed as mental illness which is mark on family. Probably not accepting of either medical or non-pharmacological treatments.

* **Self-care for symptom management.** Expectation that family members (usually women) will direct care and when possible take responsibility for symptom management. Patient can be involved if no assistance available or individual has independent personality.

Birth Rituals/Care of the New Mother/Baby

* **Pregnancy care.** Prenatal care expected if affordable. Rest encouraged. No strenuous activities. Pregnant women kept away from loud noises and from looking at people with deformities. Diet of fresh foods and low salt encouraged.

* **Labor practices.** Pregnant woman's mother present during entire labor and delivery. Although husband often discouraged from participating, involvement of husband more common among more acculturated Cubans. Physicians preferred for delivery.
* **Role of the laboring woman during birth process.** Laboring woman will assume more passive role than her mother, who will try to direct all activity. Loud expressions of pain common.
* **Role of the father and other family members during birth process.** Father's participation depends on the wife's level of acculturation and education in American cultural trends. More traditional Cuban fathers not involved at all.
* **Vaginal vs. cesarean section.** Safest procedure for mother preferred.
* **Breastfeeding.** Breastfeeding becoming more popular among Cubans.
* **Birth recuperation.** Traditionally, new mother and infant not allowed out of the home for 41 days. During this time, woman will rest and devote her energy to caring for baby. Both will be cared for by her mother and sisters. New mother will be sheltered from bad news and any stress which could harm her or the child. She will be encouraged to increase her food intake to boost milk production.
* **Problems with baby.** Any problems with baby should be discussed with woman' husband and then her mother, not directly with woman. Family will decide when information will be passed on, fearing that the mother could become hysterical and possibly have a breakdown.
* **Male and female circumcision.** Male circumcision commonly practiced. Female circumcision is not performed.

Death Rituals
* **Preparation.** Acculturated Cubans will want t be informed of their terminal illness. Less acculturated will probably follow cultural norms: first informing person directing care, male head of family and, if none, closest relative. Do not inform patient unless asked to by fam ly. Have family contact affiliated church. Entire family will be notified and expected to visit patient. Family

will wish to stay close to patient until death, including overnight.

* **Home vs. hospital.** Hospital preferred because of wish for medical treatment and pain management. Family will want all measures taken to prolong life or make patient comfortable. Receiving in-hospital medical care viewed as more important than dying at home.
* **Special needs.** Patient's family will insist on being present at all times, including overnight. Important to allow this but secure firm control over traffic. Reinforce need for rest periods for patient. Public expressions of emotion common.
* **Care of the body.** No special requirements.
* **Attitudes toward organ donation.** Organ donation not common.
* **Attitudes toward autopsy.** Autopsy not common or desired.

Family Relationships

* **Composition/structure.** Family-oriented. Extended family important. Sometimes three family generations in household. Reconstituted families still uncommon. Gay and lesbian family members usually closeted and not tolerated.
* **Decision making.** Family usually consults with most educated, respected, or eldest family member, usually male. Consultant and closest family members will then make decisions. Recommendation of MD usually followed due to importance of doctors within Cuban culture. Doctors highly respected due to education.
* **Spokesperson.** Father, eldest son or daughter, or most educated family member.
* **Gender issues.** Men expected to make decisions and protect family. Quick to show anger and aggressive behavior. Women expected to be closely involved in care and family concerns. Women usually in submissive, supportive role.
* **Caring role.** Wife, daughter, mother responsible for caring for sick family members. Patient totally submissive. Men especially will fall into helpless, dependent role. Assistance by family may hinder recovery. Education and instruction on need for self-care important.
* **Expectations of and for children.** Male children taught to be aggressive, competitive, in control, and to protect family

interest. Female children taught to be submissive, supportive, and caring. Physical punishment common. Respect of elders important. Male children exceptionally protective of mothers. Strong emphasis on and respect for education.

* **Expectations of and for elders.** Elders to be cared for by and dependent on children. Given great respect. Traditionally, family cares for elders at home until death. Elders assist in care of younger generations.

* **Expectations of adults in caring for children and elders.** Adults cared for in hospital and at home until recovery or death. Nursing homes becoming more commonly used as economic situation and acculturation influence family structure and life. Extended family will often assist when possible.

* **Expectation of visitors.** Close ties with family and friends very important in Cuban culture. Visiting sick person strong sign of respect and caring. Showing of personal and physical affection keeps connections solid.

Spiritual/Religious Orientation

* **Primary religious/spiritual affiliation.** Majority are Catholic but also many other Christian denominations represented. Those in Cuba since Castro living in a more secular state with fewer ties to church.

* **Usual religious/spiritual practices.** Praying and reciting rosary common. Worship of several important saints popular. Confession and communion important to many.

* **Use of spiritual healing/healers.** *Santaria*, an African Voodoo type religion, practiced in Cuba and among some Cubans in U.S. Sometimes when modern medicine and the church fail to heal, Cubans seek assistance from a *Santero* priest. Spells, magic, and animal sacrifices common in this practice. Sometimes specific rituals or practices must be followed or amulets must be worn. Most ceremonies will be conducted at home.

Illness Beliefs

* **Causes of physical illness.** Modern germ theory well understood. However, other causes thought possible such as

that extreme nervousness or stress can cause illness. Often illness attributed to or worsened by nerves or nervousness. Avoidance of stress, bad news, or extremes important to maintaining good health. Another possible cause of illness is evil spells or Voodoo type magic.

* **Causes of mental illness.** Mental illness is thought to be hereditary or caused by extreme stress. Mentally ill person stigmatizes family, often hidden from public or not acknowledged.

* **Causes of genetic defects.** Genetic defects explained as hereditary or due to extreme stress or trauma to mother during pregnancy. Viewing child with defect during pregnancy could also cause same defect in unborn child.

* **Sick role.** Sick person totally submissive, helpless, and dependent. May even take a passive role in decision making.

* **Home and folk remedies.** Herbal medicine often used to treat minor conditions at home.

* **Acceptance of procedures.** Procedures or interventions generally acceptable to most Cubans. Recommendations by MD are usually enough.

* **Care seeking.** First seek care from Western medical facilities. Prayer and religious assistance used concurrently. As a last resort, *Santeria* may be sought.

Health Practices

* **Concept of health.** Traditional Cubans think of someone fat (overweight) and rosy cheeked as healthy. Thin or skinny seen as poor or sickly, reflecting both socioeconomics and wasting seen in illnesses such as TB. More acculturated Cubans now accept American concepts of fitness and staying trim as healthy.

* **Health promotion and prevention.** Health promotion and illness prevention becoming more acceptable among Cubans. Medical interventions such as vaccination programs and extensive antenatal care have been vital force in health care program in Cuba under Castro. However, poor dietary habits continue to cause health problems for Cubans. Exercise not common among older community.

* **Screening.** With good education and instruc-

instruction, screening very acceptable to most.

Selected References

Hernandez, G. G. (1992). The family and its aged members: The Cuban experience. *Clinical Gerontologist, 11* (3-4), 45-57.

Pasquali, E. A. (1994). Santeria. *Journal of Holistic Nursing, 12*(4), 380-390.

Ruiz, P. (1994). Cuban Americans: Migration, acculturation, and mental health. In R.G. Malgady & O. Rodriguez (Eds.), *Theoretical and conceptual issues in Hispanic mental health* (pp. 70-89). Malabar, FL: Robert E. Krieger Publishing Co., Inc.

Author

Larry Varela, RN, MS is active in International/Cross Cultural Nursing and Community Health with emphasis on AIDS. He is a first generation Cuban-American. His parents moved to America as children, returned to Cuba after marrying, then returned back to America as refugees when Castro took power.

CHAPTER 12

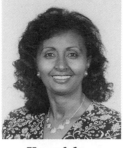

*Yewoubdar
Beyene*

Cultural/Ethnic Identity

* **Preferred terms.** Ethiopians; Eritreans.
* **History of immigration/migration.** The terms "Ethiopian" and "Eritrean" represent political entities, not separate cultural groups. Until May 1993, when a political resolution to a long-standing, bitter internal conflict divided the country, Ethiopia included Eritrea. All existing literature treats Ethiopians and Eritreans as people from the same cultural group. Ethiopia and Eritrea are multi-ethnic, multi-religious nations with many different political factions, and considerable regional variation. Despite tremendous diversity, similar core cultural values underlie behavior of most Ethiopians and Eritreans. Compared with other immigrant groups, the Ethiopian/Eritrean community in U.S. is relatively new and small. Exact size of U.S. community unknown; Ethiopians/Eritreans were subsumed in "other" or Sub-Saharan African categories for 1990 census.

1959–1970s No established Ethiopian or Eritrean community in the U.S prior to 1974. Before 1974, an estimated 3,000 Ethiopian/ Eritreans resided in U.S., 95% of whom were students and expected to return to homeland upon completion of studies. Other 5% were either diplomats or associated with various international organizations.

1975–1991 Rise to power in 1974 of Marxist Government in Ethiopia and brutal civil war in Eritrea and Tigray marked a watershed in migration pattern of Ethiopians/ Eritreans to U.S. Many residing here decided not to return home, choosing instead to seek asylum in U.S. In dramatic reversal of traditional migration patterns, majority of Ethiopians/Eritreans arriving since 1980 have come as refugees. Passage of 1980 Refugee Act enabled Africans for first time to be processed and admitted to U.S. as part of national refugee admissions ceiling established by Congress.

Most Ethiopian/Eritrean immigrants and refugees are from an urban background and live in major metropolitan U.S. cities (Washington, D.C., Los Angeles, San Francisco Bay Area, Seattle, Chicago, Dallas, Houston, Boston, and New York City), primarily on East and West Coasts. Ethiopian/Eritrean communities in U.S. are dominated by young single people with 66% males and 34% females; 70% of them are under 40 years old.

* **Map page.** *See Appendix C, p. 3.*

Communication

* **Major language(s) and dialects.** Amharic is one of the major languages in Ethiopia, and Tigrigna is national language of Eritrea. Tigrigna also major language spoken in Northern Ethiopia. In U.S., at least three major languages are spoken among Ethiopian/Eritrean immigrants/refugees: Amharic, Tigrigna, and Oromigna.
* **Literacy Assessment.** Most Ethiopians/Eritreans in the U.S. speak English: 81% have some skills—ranging from fluent to some English—but 19% have no English skills at all. Ethiopians/Eritreans speak very softly, particularly women. Elderly Ethiopians/Eritreans have minimal or no education in their own society and need assistance in translating and explaining medical procedures.
* **Nonverbal communication.** Typically very shy, polite, and reserved. Respectful to elders and authority figures (doctors and nurses). In general, little eye contact when speaking with authority figures; however, this varies based on length of time in U.S., level of education, and age and gender of individual.

People share living space, beds, etc., with other family members and friends. Touching and caressing face and hands of sick person are acceptable expressions of care, concern, and love. Touching considered healing.

Ethiopians/Eritreans often assess physicians and nurses more by warmth of manners than by professional appearance. A few opening words and show of concern and interest in patient's background will make patient feel welcome. Knowing and mentioning something, however trivial, about patient's country of origin or culture, will break the ice.

* **Use of interpreters.** Use of interpreter immensely important, not just to translate medical history and procedures but to assist health care professionals to treat patients in culturally appropriate ways. Except among large groups, most interpreters from same culture live in same community, know patient's family or friends, and cannot be neutral. Much of the time they get caught in an emotional conflict between patient and interpreter on one hand, and, on the other hand, in a cultural conflict between interpreter and health care provider, sometimes caused by health care provider's persistence in asking culturally inappropriate questions or in relating distressing information too quickly. Before communicating a serious medical situation, ask the patient if family member or close friend can be designated as spokesperson.

* **Greetings.** Hugging, kissing on cheeks, and touching are very acceptable forms of greeting among family and friends. A woman and man, or two women, kiss on cheeks three to four rounds, and hugging between men is common form of greeting. Occasionally men kiss each other on the cheeks if they are family or close friends who have not seen each other for a long time. Handshakes commonly practiced with unfamiliar people. Bowing part of formal, polite greeting of elders and authority figures. Bowing when shaking hands very common.

* **Tone of voice.** Generally soft spoken. Non-confrontational, polite. Shouting frowned on at any time. Patients and

family members rarely disagree with treatment procedures if they have placed trust in health care provider.

* **Orientation toward time.** Usually tardy in social and business situations. Difficulty in judging distance, assessing traffic, public transportation schedule, and time needed to get from place to place. Customary that Ethiopians/ Eritreans' invitation will state 6:00 p.m. for an event actually planned to start at 7:00 p.m. since guests are expected always to be late. Important to emphasize appointment time as well as medication schedule. Instead of telling patients to take their medication three or four times a day, better to be specific and say every six hours, etc.

* **Consents.** Most have no knowledge of treatment procedures and will allow physicians to decide for them. Signing consent forms written for middle-class American patient is not useful for an immigrant/refugee who has no knowledge of medical procedures; may actually induce anxiety. Informing patient about odds of not surviving the operation or the risk of dying of bleeding, anesthesia, and the like only makes patients anxious. Even though chances of an adverse outcome are statistically low, what stays with patients is negative information. Ethiopians/Eritreans gravitate to their physicians, nurses, and family for reassurance that they will make it through a crisis. Citing statistics or any evidence of a poor prognosis undercuts hope and the will to fight disease. In Ethiopia and Eritrea, consent for surgical treatment is signed by family members. U.S. health care providers should consider having a designated family member sign such papers to help alleviate anxiety in the patient.

* **Privacy.** Personal information not revealed easily, less so at first clinical encounter. Socialized to assume that it is improper to reveal oneself fully or to disclose personal secrets to anyone but a close friend. Privacy further protected by shared belief that others normally do not have just claim to information about personal matters. Reassuring confidentiality and importance of requested information for treatment plan is vital. Discuss issue with family

member or designated spokesperson to assist in choosing appropriate approaches to elicit information from the patient.

* **Serious or terminal illness.** Vital in Ethiopian/Eritrean culture to choose an appropriate time, place, and way to break bad news such as grave illness or death of a family member. Sudden shock is to be avoided at all cost because of harmful effects news may have on people with fragile emotional states. In the absence of an immediate family member, ask for a close friend. Friendship ties strong among Ethiopians/Eritreans and even stronger when they are away from their homeland. Friends substitute for extended family. In case of serious illness, health care providers communicate little information to patients. Whatever the diagnosis, they are expected to first tell bad news to family member. Family will judge how and when to let patient know. This may vary with age, level of understanding, and emotional and physical condition of sick person. In these societies, family's importance dominates individual member's right. Be selective in imparting information to family member; for example, avoid telling the mother or wife because women are socialized to be fragile.

  Communicating openly about patients' terminal illnesses evokes strong emotional reaction in patients and family, and may even interfere with care of the dying. Ethiopians/Eritreans strongly believe in destiny and in God's power to influence events, especially health events. Their persistence in holding on to hope is tied to their religious belief in God's miraculous powers.

Activities of Daily Living

* **Modesty.** Both men and women very modest. Offer hospital robes and gown. Elderly women like to wear a traditional cotton shawl on top of the gown all the time. Offer hospital pants to males when possible.
* **Skin care.** Varies by age and length of stay in U.S. Recently arrived older patients may not want to shower every day. Bathing considered relaxing, however, and even older patients will not mind showering every day if possible. Close

attention paid to hygiene and smelling good. Women like to use lotions. Some older women douche twice a day using lukewarm water only.

* **Hair care.** Women wash their hair weekly, depending on its length and texture. Those with short hair may wash twice a week. Men wash their hair each time they shower.

* **Nail care.** Men keep their nails short. Women's nail care depends on age and personal preference. Older people may object to cutting nails at night.

* **Toileting.** Will insist on using the bathroom for a) privacy; b) using bed pan uncomfortable; and c) worry about creating inconvenience for staff or family member.

* **Special clothing or amulets.** Predominantly Coptic Orthodox Christian. Allow use of religious medallions, crosses, figure of Virgin Mary or other saint, rosary beads. Moslem women may like to wear a special shawl to cover their head, may also wear amulets with Koranic verses.

* **Self-care.** Hygiene performed by patient when able. Family member or close friend may provide assistance. Women accustomed to bathing with other women and assisting each other in bathing. Older women may like to be assisted if no family member around.

Food Practices

* **Usual meal pattern.** Three times a day. Breakfast very light, lunch and dinner the major meals. Usually prefer food very spicy.

* **Special utensils.** Usual mode of eating Ethiopian/Eritrean food is with fingers; however, silverware is used for other types of food.

* **Food beliefs and rituals.** Prefer warm and soothing foods when ill—chicken or beef soups, hot oat gruel with honey, hot tea, hot milk. No ice or cold drinks.

* **Usual diet.** Usual diet consists of *enjera*, a type of bread or pancake eaten with a meat or legume sauce or stew called *wot* or *zigni*. *Enjera* made mostly from cereal called *teff*; however, a mixture of cereals can be used to make *enjera*. Legumes an important part of the diet largely prepared in the form of stew or

wot. Stew usually very spicy and contains a variety of condiments, including onions, garlic, *berbere* (hot chili powder with other spices), cardamom, white and black cumin, basil, ginger, etc. Fruits and vegetables not commonly eaten, except in some of the larger towns and during the period of religious fasting.

* **Fluids.** Generally do not drink enough water; prefer drinks at room temperature. Like to drink coffee and spice tea with cinnamon, cloves, cardamom, and lots of sugar.

* **Food prohibitions.** Considerable number of food avoidances persist among different ethnic, social, occupational, religious, age, and gender groups. Coptic Orthodox Christians and Moslems strictly observe religious taboos that forbid eating meat of wild animals, wild foul, snakes, wild and domestic pigs, dogs, horses, and shellfish. Coptic Christians do not eat meat or dairy for 200 days of each year.

* **Food prescriptions.** Preferences are chicken or beef soups, noodles and pasta, traditional hot oat gruel with honey. Do not like bland foods.

Symptom Management

* **Pain.** Stoic, with high pain threshold. Patients do not explain symptoms clearly; hard to pinpoint symptoms, very general; no understanding of numerical scale of expressing pain. Do not like pain medication because of concern about addiction. Older women usually moan to express pain, act very helpless and passive.

* **Dyspnea.** Will hyperventilate and panic. Family members also panic and hover over the sick person. Will use oxygen; however, need reassurance since using oxygen and any other major intervention is associated with gravity of disease. Also explain to family members necessity for oxygen, since their panic increases patient's anxiety level.

* **Nausea/vomiting.** May alert family member or RN before vomiting and ask for medication. Tendency to clean up or throw away vomitus. Explain to patient and family caregiver about waiting for RN before throwing away vomitus. Traditionally lemon peel, ginger root, rue, or fennel used to control nausea.

*   **Constipation/diarrhea.** Will only disclose
    when asked. Traditional remedies for
    constipation include herbs, castor oil,
    epsom salts, or some form of laxative.
    For diarrhea, eating rice or drinking
    rice water recommended. Dehydration
    associated with diarrhea not recognized
    so patient should be encouraged to
    drink fluid.

*   **Fatigue.** Older people like taking naps after
    lunch. Overall, very hesitant to accept
    sleeping pills for fear of strong effect
    and future dependency.

*   **Depression.** Ethiopians'/Eritreans' patterns of
    somatization of anxiety and depression
    and negative attitudes toward psychia-
    try are similar to those of immigrants
    from the Middle East. Resist seeking
    help from mental health counselors
    because of cultural stigma associated
    with mental illness. Deny any relation-
    ship between worries and vague com-
    plaints for which no physical cause
    can be found. Somatization a way of
    coping with original anxiety. (See
    also Privacy).

*   **Self-care for symptom management.** Delay
    seeking professional help. Use home
    remedies and other means, and do not
    seek medical care until in severe pain.
    Do not like to go to physician for rou-
    tine examination.

Birth Rituals/Care of the New Mother/Baby

*   **Pregnancy care.** Traditionally, pregnancy con-
    sidered a dangerous state, as fetus could
    be easy prey for evil eye and sorcery
    believed to cause miscarriage, prema-
    ture delivery, and fetal malformation.
    Expectant mother given much
    attention by her family and others,
    supposed to avoid excesses in com-
    monplace activities: carrying heavy
    loads, climbing stairs, and exposure to
    emotional situations such as funerals,
    fights, bad news. Encouraged to eat
    well, get plenty of sleep, and avoid
    day-to-day tasks that require bending
    and lifting. Craving for particular food
    given special attention. Generally
    believed that unfulfilled craving will
    cause miscarriage. Walking and mov-
    ing around are encouraged as due date
    gets closer. Traditionally, pregnant
    woman drinks a hot mixture of ground
    toasted flax seed and water sweetened
    with honey or sugar (mixture believed

to ease labor or as laxative) a week
before due date.

* **Labor practices.** Traditionally a self-trained
midwife or an older female family
member assists with delivery. In urban
areas, women are accustomed to hospital delivery. Overall, tolerate labor
pain; prefer presence of female family
members and friends who provide
comfort, massage her back and feet.
Women may hesitate to take pain
medication.

* **Role of the laboring woman during birth
process.** Woman takes an active role
during labor; modesty very important
so needs to be kept covered. Low level
of moaning or grunting socially acceptable; however, screaming socially unacceptable.

* **Role of the father and other family members
during birth process.** Traditionally,
father and male family members not
allowed to be with birthing woman.
In U.S., however, young fathers participate in Lamaze and stay close to wives
during delivery.

* **Vaginal vs. cesarean section.** Vaginal
delivery preferred.

* **Breastfeeding.** Traditionally, mothers breast
feed for an average of 23 months or
more; no taboo against breastfeeding
in public. Overall, women prefer
breastfeeding as much as possible;
however, in U.S., working mothers use
formula along with breastfeeding.
Women eat special foods and drink
milk and gruel made from oats and
honey to increase their breast milk.

* **Birth recuperation.** New mother expected to
be with baby 24 hours a day. Female
family members assist new mother in
bathing and caring for baby. Both
mother and baby are considered deli-
cate and every effort is made to protect
them from disease and harm. At least
40 days seclusion is prescribed for
mother and baby. Mother is fed special
foods: porridge made from barley and
other cereals, meat, and chicken stew,
etc. Her food and drinks must be
warm. Childbirth considered a joyful
event and received by family and
neighbors with joyous food sharing and
gift giving to mother and baby.

* **Problems with baby.** If problem with baby,
best to consult with father or other
family member. Do not tell mother or

any immediate female family members. Ask spokesperson for advice.

* **Male and female circumcision.** Among Christians male circumcision traditionally done eight days after birth. In urban settings, however, and in U.S., it is common to allow new baby boys to be circumcised before discharge. Female circumcision and clitoridectomy practiced throughout homeland. However, this tradition varies, based on regional practices, urban/rural settings, religion, and level of parental education. Most urban and educated families in Ethiopian/Eritrea do not follow these traditions. Most common procedure among Christians is excision of prepuce performed seven days after birth. This practice not perceived as an initiation or rite of passage, but carried out in infancy, almost before child is given an identity. Varying with area, social class, religion, and education, infibulation (removal of labia minora clitoris and sewing of labia majora—leaving a small hole for urination and menstruation) practiced among Moslems.

Death Rituals
* **Preparation.** Culturally important how tragic news is communicated (see Serious or terminal illness). News of death of family member is disclosed to close friends before family is told so that friends will be there to provide emotional support. Never tell female family member first. Spokesperson may arrange for a Coptic priest (where available) or religious figure for patient to receive sacrament.
* **Home vs. hospital.** Traditionally, people prefer loved one to die at home; in U.S., however, prefer patient to stay in hospital. (Ethiopian/Eritrean immigrant community in U.S. mostly young urban people whereas tradition of dealing with death usually domain of older people.)
* **Special needs.** Ethiopian/Eritrean culture restrains most emotional outburst except at death of loved ones when great demonstrations of feeling are encouraged. They cry loudly and uncontrollably. Women tear their clothes and beat their chests until the

become sick with grief. Men permitted to cry out loud and shed tears.

* **Care of the body.** Ethiopian/Eritrean community in U.S. accept standard procedure of preparing body at morgue. Some family members may want to say good-bye prior to body's being taken to morgue; not customary and may vary among families. Throughout the homeland, people bury their dead. Cremation not unacceptable unless specified.

* **Attitudes toward organ donation.** Idea of organ donation new to this group. Check with family members.

* **Attitudes toward autopsy.** Autopsy unacceptable unless family is convinced is medically necessary.

Family Relationships

* **Composition/structure.** Extended family most important institution. However, in U.S. community of mostly young single people, close friends substitute for extended family. Typical household of Ethiopians/Eritreans in U.S. consists of siblings, cousins, and friends. Common in these groups to introduce childhood friend or very close friend as sibling. Gay and lesbian family members are not acknowledged.

* **Decision making.** Family members work as a unit. Traditionally, father or oldest son has leading role. However, in U.S., even if father is living with family, lead role in decision making is given to most acculturated family member.

* **Spokesperson.** Father, oldest son, or daughter. However, in U.S., most acculturated family member becomes spokesperson.

* **Gender issues.** Mostly men are expected to make decisions, particularly at time of family crisis. Men in charge of breaking bad news, making funeral arrangements, religious services, taking care of financial needs, etc.

* **Caring role.** Women are major caregivers. Female family members (mothers, grandmothers, sisters, cousins) or close friends expected to care for sick. However, in absence of close female family member, husbands and brothers provide care. During illness and crisis, Ethiopians/Eritreans rely heavily on family members to help them cope. Patient pampered with attention and services, protected from emotional

upsets. Caregivers do not encourage
patient to be independent.
Ambulation must be stressed
and reinforced.

* **Expectations of and for children.** Infancy is
prolonged and indulged; children
raised in highly protective environment. From about three years on, child
is subjected to regime of discipline.
Obedience and politeness are overrid-
ing goals of bringing up children.
Physical aggression discouraged; quiet,
reserved manner of speaking emphasized. Children who are noisy and disrespectful considered rude. Strong
emphasis on education.

* **Expectations of and for elders.** Elders respected and looked after by their children.
Children remain deeply attached to
families and sensitive to wishes of parents. Children responsible for taking
care of their old parents. Elders play
major role in raising and disciplining
grandchildren.

* **Expectations of adults in caring for children
and elders.** Adults responsible for caring for sick family member.
Traditionally, elders are cared for at
home; nursing home or hospice unacceptable option.

* **Expectation of visitors.** Friends and family
members constantly come to visit sick
person throughout the day. Even when
patient is too sick to interact, people
feel they must be there in support of
family at difficult times. Ethiopian/
Eritrean patients do not like to be left
alone. Family and friends want to stay
at bedside at all times. In grave illness
situation, family and friends like to
stay overnight with patient in hospital.

Spiritual/Religious Orientation

* **Primary religious/spiritual affiliation.**
Predominantly Coptic Orthodox
Christian. A few Catholics and
Protestants. Many Moslems in eastern
region of Ethiopian and in Eritrea.

* **Usual religious/spiritual practices.** Families
may say prayers, read the Bible, rub
patient's forehead and body with holy
water. Older patients may like visit
from priest.

* **Use of spiritual healing/healers.** No traditional Ethiopian/Eritrean healers in
U.S. Healing tradition usually domain
of older people and religious leaders.

Illness Beliefs

*   **Causes of physical illness.** Ethiopians/
    Eritreans have two broad etiological
    theories of disease: naturalistic and
    magico-religious. Diseases more often
    diagnosed in naturalistic rather than in
    magico-religious category. In naturalis-
    tic etiology, sickness may result from
    external factors, such as drinking pol-
    luted water, eating unfamiliar or
    spoiled food, contagion, interpersonal
    conflict, personal excess (i.e., emotion-
    al distress, etc.). In magico-religious
    etiology, illnesses attributed to God,
    nature and demonic spirits, magical
    forces, or breach of social taboos or
    personal vows.
*   **Causes of mental illness.** Traditionally, ail-
    ments such as mental illness and
    epilepsy routinely attributed to action
    of evil spirits.
*   **Causes of genetic defects.** Accepted as will of
    God. Family members expected to care
    for child at home. Institutionalization
    frowned on.
*   **Sick role.** Sick person acts helpless, passive,
    totally dependent on family members.
    Family and friends expected to look
    after the sick, prepare food, clean up
    after, and pamper. Customary to bring
    home cooked, soothing foods to
    patient. Family members alter their
    schedules to attend needs of sick.
*   **Home and folk remedies.** Self-care by house-
    holds without use of professional heal-
    ers common throughout Ethiopia and
    Eritrea. Their pharmacopeia largely
    derivatives from the natural world:
    plants, grains, spices, oil seeds, herbs,
    butter. Popular remedies against
    headaches include coffee and lemon
    tea; boiling or smelling eucalyptus
    leaves used to treat cold. In U.S. most
    Ethiopians/Eritreans rely on Western
    biomedicine.
*   **Acceptance of procedures.** Explain proce-
    dures clearly to patient and family
    members. Patient and family members
    rarely disagree with treatment proce-
    dures if they trust health care provider.
    Fearful of surgery, and of donating or
    receiving blood. However, this varies,
    based on age and length of stay in U.S.
*   **Care seeking.** Ethiopians/Eritreans in U.S.
    do not have folk healers but rely

mainly on biomedicine. However, there are some illnesses for which they feel folk medicine is better, and some go to their homeland for treatment. Community generally resistant to psychiatric treatment.

Health Practices

* **Concept of health.** Health defined as state of equilibrium among physiological, spiritual, cosmological, ecological, and social forces surrounding humans. Well-being thought to be secured by peaceful relationship with supernatural world.

* **Health promotion and prevention.** Proper function of human body viewed as being dependent on physiological balance and adequate food intake. Eating and drinking moderately, avoiding emotional distress, never bathing in cold water, avoiding exposure to atmospheric changes, and cleanliness thought to promote health.

* **Screening.** In Ethiopian/Eritrean culture, patient-healer relationship is paternalistic and protective, and trust a major component of relationship. Screening poses no problem; however, modesty could be an issue.

Selected References

Beyene, Y. (1992). Medical disclosure and refugees: Telling bad news to Ethiopian patients. *Western Journal of Medicine, 157*(3), 328-332.

Kloos, H. & Zein, A.Z. (Eds.) (1993). *The ecology of health and disease in Ethiopia.* Boulder, CO: Westview Press.

Levin, D.N. (1965). *Wax and gold: Tradition and innovation in Ethiopian culture* (5th Ed.). Chicago, IL: University of Chicago Press.

Author

Yewoubdar Beyene, PhD is Assistant Research Anthropologist in the Medical Anthropology Program of the Department of Epidemiology and Biostatistics at the University of California, San Francisco. Born and raised in Ethiopia, she came to U.S. in 1972 as a master's student. She studies immigrants and refugees and cross-cultural perspectives on menopause.

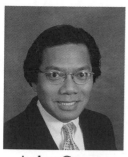

Arthur Cantos

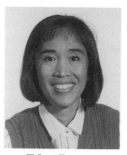

Eden Rivera

Cultural/Ethnic Identity

* **Preferred terms.** Filipino-American—accepted English spelling. Pilipino-American—correct spelling (no F in Pilipino alphabet).

* **History of immigration.**

First Wave:

Early 1700s Manila men deserted Spanish galleons in Mexico, emigrated to New Orleans, Louisiana.

1906–1934 Manong generation, male agricultural workers to Hawaii and western U.S.

1934 Tydings-McDuffie Act made Philippines a commonwealth. Annual quota = 50 Filipinos.

Second Wave:

1946–1965 Citizenship to Filipinos who joined the armed services in WWII, recruits, war brides, students, and professionals.

Third Wave:

1965 Amended Immigration Naturalization Act of 1934 relaxed quotas, bringing in large proportion of young professionals, unskilled laborers, and families.

* **Map page.** *See Appendix C, p. 4.*

Communication

* **Major language and dialects.** Pilipino (Tagalog) is the national language. There are 85 major languages and dialects. Most common dialects are *Ilocano*, *Cebuano*, *Bicolano*, *Pampango*, and *Chabacano*. English the language of choice in schools, businesses, and mass media. Most Filipinos speak English with a distinctive accent.

* **Literacy assessment.** Most Filipinos speak and understand English. Remember to speak slowly. Filipinos are sensitive to the tone and manner of speaker.

Use simple medical terminologies.

Elderly Filipinos minimal or no education may need assistance with reading or writing English.

* **Nonverbal communication.** Typically shy and affectionate. Awkward in unfamiliar surroundings. Respectful to elders and authority figures (nurses and doctors). Touching not uncommon. Little direct eye contact, particularly with superiors and authority figures.

  Personal space is constricted, frequently shared with other family members. Allow a family member to stay at bedside at all times. May be reluctant to venture out of personal space or leave room for any reason.

  Polite. Will tend not to disagree. Assess meaning of silence, whether as approval or not. Handshakes not commonly practiced.

* **Use of interpreters.** Include family members in translation. For privacy reasons, discuss sensitive issues such as sex, diagnosis or prognosis, and socioeconomic status with close family member.

* **Greetings.** Filipinos smile a lot, whether as greeting or as acknowledgment. Can be animated, using facial expression such as a smile and raised eyebrows instead of a verbal response. Elderly people are shown respect by kissing hand, forehead, or cheeks.

* **Tone of voice.** Filipino language as a practical language is not very rich. Instead, Filipinos change the tone of voice to emote or to romanticize the language.

  Can get loud in the presence of a group of family members. May get agitated or emotional when nervous or frightened.

  As a sign of respect, the use of *po* and *opo* is added in the sentence. *Saan po masakit?* = "where does it hurt?"

  Uncomfortable giving commands prefer to request politely. Typically so spoken, Filipinos avoid direct expression of disagreements.

* **Orientation towards time.** Both past and present orientation. Filipino time usually means being tardy in social settings. Business time is followed for medical appointments, church, and work. Because of several clocks, emphasize importance of keeping appointments and medication schedule.

Bahala na (God willing) is a fatalistic outlook on life whereby a person believes that one should unquestioningly accept what life and death bring. This attitude influences Filipinos' time orientation.

* **Consents.** Explain procedures or surgical intervention clearly. Stop frequently to elicit feedback from patients or allow questions; otherwise patient will be uncomfortable asking questions.

* **Privacy.** Sensitive to concept of shame (*Hiya*) or saving face. Strong respect for authority will allow disclosure of private information if relevant to care. Include close family members when necessary, particularly if patient requests their presence.

* **Serious or terminal illness.** See *Bahala Na*, above.

   Do not tell the patient without consulting the family or at least the eldest son or daughter. Allow patient's family to disclose the prognosis. The presence of an MD, RN, or a social worker may be requested.

Activities of Daily Living

* **Modesty.** Very modest, particularly the women. Offer hospital robe plus hospital gown. Offer hospital pants to male patients.

* **Skin care.** Prefer to shower daily, if no surgical incisions or invasive tubes. Pay close attention to hygiene and smelling good. Thorough peri care; some prefer soap and water peri wash after every BM or urination (female).

* **Hair care.** Prefer to wash hair daily.

* **Nail care.** No cutting at night.

* **Toileting.** Will insist on using the bathroom for two reasons: privacy, and to do a thorough peri wash using soap and water.

* **Special clothing/amulets.** Predominantly Catholic. Allow use of religious medallions, rosary beads, or a figure of a saint.

* **Self-care.** Hygiene will be performed by the patient when able. A family member may be able to provide assistance. If no family member is around, maintain privacy and modesty.

Food Practices

* **Usual meal pattern.** Meal times—3 times a day. Snacks in between meals.

* **Food beliefs and rituals.** Prefers soft and warm food when ill. No ice in drinks.
* **Usual diet.** Rice with every meal. Enjoy fish, meat, and vegetables. Like fried food. Add salt to food on the table, or soy or fish sauce to enhance the flavor. Think American cuisine is bland. Like food with sauce or broth
* **Fluids.** Drink a lot of water, at room temperature or warmer.
* **Food prohibitions.** Some Filipinos have lactose intolerance and difficulty digesting wheat bread. Some devout Catholics prefer not to eat meat on Fridays, especially during Lent. No extremely cold or acidic food (orange juice, fresh chilled fruits) first thing in the morning.
* **Food prescriptions.** Enjoy rice porridge when ill. Ask dietary kitchen for Asian or Chinese menu, when available.

Symptom Management
* **Pain.** (*Masakit*) Can be stoic. Offer pain meds, as ordered. Some have high pain threshold. Understand numerical scale of expressing pain. Fearful of becoming addicted to narcotics. Hate IM, prefer P.O. or IV. Offer warm compress when necessary. Some will moan as a way of expressing pain.
* **Dyspnea.** (*Hindi makahinga*—can't breath) Get frantic when dyspneic. Will hyperventilate. Will use oxygen after some explanation. Some will be more anxious about using oxygen, associating its use with increasing gravity of disease.
* **Nausea/vomiting.** (*Nasusuka*—nauseated) Because of modesty and shame, will alert RN after vomiting. Some will clean up or throw away vomitus. Some will ask RN for nausea medication.
* **Constipation/diarrhea.** Become uncomfortable if routine BM is disrupted. Will only disclose this to RN when asked (modesty). Will accept measures to correct alteration in bowel functions. Enema only as last resort.
* **Fatigue.** (*Pagod*—tired) Naps in early afternoon. Hesitant to use sleeping pills for fear of addiction.
* **Depression.** (*Lungkot*—sad) Because of shame, will not acknowledge to RN unless asked.
* **Self-care for symptom management.** Does not respond to illness until advanced, is taken to bed, or is in severe pain.

Birth Rituals/Care of the New Mother/Baby

*   **Pregnancy care.** Prenatal care an expectation for those who can afford it. Family gives much attention to the pregnant woman. She is not allowed to work outside the home. She is encouraged to eat well and is given choice foods when possible. She is encouraged to get plenty of sleep at night. In the last few months, she is discouraged from staying in a dependent position, such as prolonged sitting or sleeping during the day for fear of water retention. Sexual intercourse is taboo during the last two months of pregnancy.

    As the time of birth draws near, the traditional Filipino woman is encouraged to eat fresh eggs based on the belief that eating slippery foods will allow the baby to "slip" through the birth canal.

*   **Labor practices.** If an MD is not present during labor, a self-trained "midwife" assists with delivery. Noise and stimulation are minimized for fear that too much commotion will increase labor pains. Father usually not with the wife during labor, unless Lamaze is being practiced. Some fathers remain at work or with their male friends for support.

    Some pregnant woman may try to walk around the room to promote dilatation. Offer adequate pain relief; some may refuse.

*   **Role of laboring woman during birth process.** The soon-to-be-mother assumes an active role during labor, sometimes commanding either the family or the midwife to cover or fan her. Most women will keep moaning or grunting to an accepted social level. Others may scream and become hysterical.

*   **Role of the father and other family members during birth process.** The father assumes a passive role during the birth process, except for those who attend Lamaze classes. A female member of the family who is a mother is preferred to be the coach during labor.

*   **Vaginal vs. caesarean section.** Vaginal delivery is preferred.

*   **Breastfeeding.** Breast feeding is an expectation of all Filipino mothers, sometimes until the child is a toddler. For working mothers, breastfeeding is

concurrently practiced with formula feeding until the child is at least a year old. Some seafood, i.e., clams and fish, is avoided for unknown reasons.

* **Birth recuperation.** The new mother is expected to be with the baby 24 hours a day. Most of the new tasks are shared by the mother and a sister and the father. The mother is freed from heavy housework, provided with nourishing soup to drink, and pampered with attention.

    While recuperating, the mother is encouraged to use a pelvic binder for at least six weeks. New mothers discouraged from showering immediately; however, hygiene is of utmost importance. Mothers may give themselves a thorough sponge bath, sometimes many times in a day. Peri care is done by washing with soap and water, or by adding some drops of vinegar to the warm water.

* **Problems with the baby.** If there is a problem with the baby, it is best to consult with the father and other family support, such as the mother of the new mother, prior to informing her. The MD must be the person telling the new mother.

* **Male and female circumcision.** Male circumcision not traditionally done at birth. However, for working parents, it is now common practice to allow their new baby boy to be circumcised prior to discharge. Female circumcision never performed.

Death Rituals

* **Preparation.** Inform head of family (usually parents or eldest children) away from patient's room. Notify Catholic chaplain for patient to receive Sacrament of the Sick. Do not resuscitate (DNR) is usually a very difficult choice; will be decided by entire family.

* **Home vs. hospital.** If diagnosis is terminal for chronic illness, will prefer to die at home with dignity. Arrange for hospice set up. For acute illness, will prefer for patient to stay in the hospital.

* **Special needs.** May ask for religious medallions, rosary beads, and other objects of spiritual significance, such as a figurine of a saint, to be near the patient. Family may start praying at the bedside for a dying family member.

May start crying loudly and uncontrollably, even hysterically.

* **Care of body.** Death given very high regard—a spiritual event. Family may want to wash the body. Will want all the family members to say good-bye prior to body being taken down to morgue.
* **Attitude toward organ donation.** The body is given high respect. Cremation is not a common practice. May not allow organ donation.
* **Attitudes toward autopsy.** Same as above. If medically necessary, entire family will decide.

Family Relationships

* **Composition and structure.** Family oriented cultural group. Both extended and nuclear family. Sometimes three family generations in a household. Tolerant and supportive of gay or lesbian sibling.
* **Decision making.** Father or eldest son acts as the family spokesperson; however, decisions usually made by entire family.
* **Spokesperson.** Father, eldest son, or daughter.
* **Gender issues.** Men expected to make decisions or arrangements such as transferring patient back to house or other care facility or calling the mortuary. Women act as primary bedside care providers regardless of whether patient is male or female.
* **Caring role.** Women, mother or a responsible daughter, even a niece or other female relative are expected to care for the sick. Patient is pampered with attention and services, sometimes hindering in care, particularly with ambulation and self-care activities.
* **Expectations of and for children.** Children reared in a highly protective environment. Emphasis on negative sanctions versus positive rewards by means of frightening, teasing, and shaming to avoid possible misconduct. For example, "If you go out of your room, the boogie man will get you." Taught to be quiet and avoid direct confrontations about personal differences, to contain emotions, and to be obedient, respectful, and shy.

    Strong emphasis on education, particularly college education. Education means material and personal gain.

* **Expectations of and for elders.** Elders given due respect. Tone of voice during conversation is softer. When elders become ill, children will be expected to care for them, returning all the favors afforded them.

  Depending on socioeconomic status, elders sometimes care for their grandchildren to allow employed members of family to earn a living.

* **Expectations of adults caring for children and elders.** Adults to care for sick or injured until health is regained or eventual death. Traditionally, sick elders are cared for at home; however, in higher socioeconomic group where all family members are either at work or in school, sick or frail elder person is placed in a nursing home with much emotional difficulty. Some Filipinos believe such an act is disrespectful to a parent.

* **Expectations of visitors.** Female family member may stay at bedside for duration of patient's hospital stay. Offer a private room, give family a quick orientation of the unit, such as showing them location of pantry, linen, cafeteria, and chapel.

  Because Filipinos are family oriented, entire family may come to visit the sick.

Spiritual/Religious Orientation

* **Primary religious/spiritual affiliation.** Predominantly Catholic. Some Protestants and Moslems (from the southern part of the country).

* **Usual religious/spiritual practices.** Religious family may recite the rosary or read novena prayers. Call for chaplain to visit, whether for confession, communion, or receiving the sacrament of the sick.

* **Use of spiritual healing/healers.** In the Philippines, when one becomes ill a physician, as well as a priest, is summoned. Very important for patient to see a priest, particularly if terminally ill.

Illness Beliefs

* **Causes of physical illness.** Health is a result of balance (*timbang*). Illness is the result of some imbalance. Some associate illness with bad behavior or

punishment, and to become healthy again is to correct the evil deed.

Filipinos often do not respond to illness until it is quite advanced and patient is taken to bed, suffering from severe pain, or lapses into unconsciousness. The basic logic of health and illness involves both prevention (avoidance of inappropriate behaviors that cause imbalance) and curing (by restoring balance).

* **Causes of mental illness.** Catholicism and mystical causation beliefs coexist in the same person. Mental illness occurs when there is disruption of harmonious function of whole individual and spiritual world.

    Mystical, contact with person or with stronger life force. **Supernatural,** life force in all objects manifesting as ghost (*multo*) or souls of dead. **Naturalistic**, wind, vapors, diet, shifted bodily organs and stress. **Western,** physical and emotional strain, sexual frustration, unrequited love and inherited constitutional defects.

* **Causes of genetic defects.** Filipinos are accepting of their loved ones' genetic defects believing it the will of God or punishment for bad behavior. Will tend to care for child at home rather than institutionalize.

* **Sick role.** A sick member of the family is treated well. It is the expectation of the sick to have a family member looking after him/her, to bring food from home that is soothing for the body, i.e., rice soup. The patient assumes a passive role where decisions are made for him/her.

* **Home and folk remedies.** Because of Chinese influence in the culture, some Filipinos use herbal medicine prior to seeking medical help. Some believe that every physical ailment is caused by the supernatural. In hospital, Filipinos tend to rely on Western medicine and care.

* **Acceptance of procedures.** Explain procedures clearly and slowly. Some Filipinos more fearful of donating blood than receiving blood. Donating blood is thought to cause an imbalance in health. Family may want to donate blood only for loved ones.

* **Care seeking.** Filipinos believe concurrently in modern medicine and folk

diagnosticians. Certain conditions believed to worsen from western bio-medical treatment. Some believe in the role of healers who can placate or exorcise spirits and ghosts.

Health Practices

* **Concept of health.** Good health related to maintaining balance. Associate health with good food, freedom from pain, and strength. Being overweight not a concern, instead seen as sign of good socioeconomic standing and contentment.

* **Health promotion and prevention.** To promote health is to maintain balance. Eating well, not necessarily eating right, thought to promote good health. Keeping oneself clean looking and smelling promotes good health. Optimal health maintained by keeping warm. Exercise not a regular part of Filipinos' activities of daily living. Ambulation and pulmonary toilet after surgery has to be stressed and reinforced. To prevent illness is to avoid behavior that causes imbalance.

* **Screening.** Filipinos have great respect towards medical authority. Screening, if properly asked with due respect to modesty issues, will pose no problem, except in the area of sex and a diagnosis with a poor prognosis. Most will disclose their medical diagnosis and pertinent information related to the disease process.

    Be sure to ask family regarding home setting. The family is a very strong support to any Filipino, sick or not.

Selected References

Anderson, J. N. (1983). Health and illness in Pilipino immigrants. *Western Journal of Medicine, 139,* 811-819.

Espiritu, Y. (1995). *Filipino American lives.* Philadelphia: Temple University Press.

Orque, M. S. (1983). Nursing care of Filipino American patients. In M. S. Orque, B. Block, & L. S. A. Monrroy (Eds.), *Ethnic nursing care - A multicultural approach* (pp. 149-181). St. Louis, MO: C. V. Mosby Co.

Wilson, S., & Billones, H. (1994). The Filipino elder: Implications for nursing practice. *Journal of Gerontological Nursing, 20*(8), 31-36.

Authors

Arthur D. Cantos, RN, BSN is an assistant nurse manager at UCSF Medical Center - Cardiothoracic/ Vascular Surgeries and Cardiology Unit. Born in the Philippines, Arthur is the Chairman of the Filipino Community Heart Council of the American Heart Association in San Francisco and speaks on "Eating Smart, Filipino Style."

Eden Rivera, RN, BSN is acting nurse manager of the liver transplant, general surgery, urology and otolaryngology unit at UCSF Medical Center. She wishes to acknowledge her parents who were born in the Philippines, emigrated to the U.S. a year before Eden was born, and continued to instill in their children an appreciation of the Pilipino culture by practicing traditional customs and cooking traditional foods.

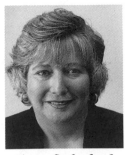

Anne Sutherland

Cultural/Ethnic Identity

* **Preferred terms.** There are many different Gypsy groups with diverse cultural practices. Most groups recognize the term Gypsy as used by non-Gypsies. Largest group of Gypsies in U.S. call themselves *Roma* (sing. *Rom*).

* **History of immigration.** Records of Gypsies in U.S. date from 1600s (mainly English Gypsies), but largest immigration was from 1880s to beginning of 20th century. In 1920s and 1930s, Gypsies migrated from East Coast to West Coast. Many came to U.S. through South America and some through Canada.

Communication

* **Major language(s) and dialects.** Romanes (Romany) is first language, but all Gypsies in U.S. speak English. Often they have a strong accent (e.g., pronounce w for v) or interchange words that sound alike (world's fair for welfare). Depending on individual's country of origin, will also speak language of that area (Russian, Greek, Serbian, Spanish).

* **Literacy assessment.** Older Gypsies have no formal education and are unable to read and write other than to sign their name. Need to read important documents to them rather than ask if they can read as they are sensitive about illiteracy, or ask if there is younger family member who can read aloud to patient. Not all younger Gypsies can read, however. May appear to understand medical terminology when they do not; need to confirm understanding.

* **Nonverbal communication.** Often gregarious and assertive, appearing aggressive or even threatening, one way to show

their concern over illness. Can alternate mood quickly from aggressive to begging for help. Facial expressions may reflect suspicion. First reaction often mistrustful; important to take time to establish trust.

Very respectful of elders' authority. Appeal to eldest person present to keep order with others. Respectful of older medical personnel, but may dismiss younger medical personnel as too young to know anything. Bring in older professional with young doctor to establish authority.

Desire close personal contact with family members. Allow family member to stay in room at all times. Very anxious when alone.

Gypsies avoid close contact with non-Gypsies and impure surfaces (e.g., toilet, bathrooms, floor, areas where lower body has touched).

* **Use of interpreters.** Use younger family members for translation and explanation of terms.
* **Greetings.** Greet each other by raising hand palm up and calling out *baXt hai sastimos* (luck and health). Normally very animated, but in illness become very anxious (in English they say "my nerves").
* **Tone of voice.** Very loud and argumentative as matter of course. Does not always mean they are arguing. Shouting a common form of teasing and joking, even an affectionate form of communication. Real anger does erupt; however, usually contained by family members. Gypsies very rarely violent. Best not to overreact.

Grief expressed by wailing and calling out to God (*Devla...*) over and over. Women may beat their breasts and tear out hair. Also a fear reaction to death (spirit of dead person may haunt them).

* **Orientation toward time.** Generally not time oriented as they do not go to school or hold jobs. Understand appointment times perfectly well, but often fail to show up unless aware of importance.
* **Consents.** Explain procedures clearly and ask for feedback from patient. Do not underestimate intelligence and abili to grasp complex procedures, but m sure that one or two unfamiliar wo have not led to misunderstanding.

Cancer associated with certain death; need to explain risk immediately. Patient can sign written consent after verbal explanation.

* **Privacy.** Men and women extremely modest regarding procedures dealing with lower body, women more so than men. Examinations of lower body very sensitive as are discussion of body fluids (menstrual blood, urine, feces). Shame and embarrassment associated with these topics. Upper body/body fluids hold no shame or embarrassment. Women sometimes pinch each other's breasts to show affection, for example. Vomit and spittle not viewed as dirty or shameful.

  Ask for personal information only in presence of family member of same sex, never in mixed company.

* **Serious or terminal illness.** Best to have doctor in authority tell of serious illness or death. Tell closest, oldest relatives first and ask them to inform rest of family. Carefully choose time to inform as news will create crisis.

  Gypsies express grief very openly and view serious illness as major group crisis and tragedy for patient and family. Although more accepting of death at old age or death for which they have been prepared, death of young person not accepted but fought against strongly. News of illness and death travels rapidly throughout community gathered together for crisis. Best to provide space for large numbers of people to gather and grieve (e.g., a garden area) rather than try to keep them out.

Activities of Daily Living

* **Modesty.** Very modest in regard to lower body. Offer clean robe plus gown and pants for men. Examinations of men should be done by men, of women by women. Sex separation very important.
* **Skin care.** Prefer to keep skin moist; offer cream. Hygiene viewed as essential to moral character. Hygiene consists of keeping lower body separate from upper body. Offer separate towels and soaps for each half of body. Allow frequent hand washing.
* **Hair care.** Head symbolically important to keep clean by keeping away anything from rest of body. Men particularly must keep their heads "pure." Provide

clean pillowcases when possible. Try not to touch head or pillowcase.

* **Nail care.** Hands washed frequently. Feet must be kept separate. Sterilize nail cutter used for feet before offering for hands.

* **Toileting.** Prefer toileting in privacy. If bedpan necessary, have person of same sex as patient help and keep bedpan away from upper body.

* **Special clothing/amulets.** Most Gypsies wear an amulet around neck (especially children). Allow amulet under pillow or at bedside table. Never put amulet at foot of bed. Man's hat and woman's scarf also must be kept by head and not at foot of bed.

* **Self-care.** Allow patient and patient's family to provide care when possible. Family members very attentive. Long term self-care is problematic as Gypsies often stop medication when they feel better. Explain importance of taking full course of medications.

Food Practices

* **Usual meal pattern.** Three meals a day, largest at lunch and dinner. Light breakfast or just coffee.

* **Special utensils.** No silverware, only disposable plastic utensils. Prefer to use hands if they can wash before meal.

* **Food beliefs and rituals.** Food must be prepared in way that is "clean" (wrapped in plastic, on paper plates, or anything disposable). Will avoid eating anything presented on plates that must be washed.

* **Usual diet.** Heavy and greasy, high in salt and cholesterol. Eat white bread with every meal. Prefer barbecued meat and salad with lots of dressing. Usual diet related to many commonly found illness among Gypsies, such as diabetes, hemorrhoids, hypertension, and heart disease.

* **Fluids.** Drink a lot of coffee, sweet tea, beer, and cokes.

* **Food prohibitions.** Some Gypsies prefer fish on Fridays. Some fast on Fridays or avoid animal products (meat, eggs, lard, butter). Relatives of sick person sometimes fast and/or avoid animal products to help sick person recove

    Will not eat food that has bee handled too much by non-Gypsie food comes with a cover, allow p to remove cover. Generally believed that eating impure food causes illness.

Breastfeeding mothers avoid greens (e.g., cabbage), pickled foods, and tomatoes.

When someone dies, sour foods are shunned (sour cream, lemons, or vinegar).

* **Food prescriptions.** Certain foods promote luck and good health. Garlic, black pepper, red pepper, salt, vinegar, onions, and pickled foods viewed as especially healthy, used as cures for illnesses and often in amulets around neck or sewn into clothes.

Symptom Management

* **Pain.** Will describe pain willingly but accurate knowledge of anatomy lacking so nonspecific terms used to locate pain. Avoid rectal administration of pain meds. Oral or IV route preferred. Adults not stoic and moan loudly; children more stoic. Numerical pain scale understood.

* **Dyspnea.** Prone to excitement and hyperventilation. Use of oxygen usually accepted, but general fear of anesthesia (referred to as "little death"). Oxygen mask may be mistaken for anesthesia.

* **Nausea/vomiting.** Will readily report nausea or vomiting. No prohibitions on vomiting. One of their most powerful medicines is "ghost's vomit."

* **Constipation/diarrhea.** Will avoid discussing diarrhea. Constipation and hemorrhoids very common problems because of diet; may need help with constipation. Use of enemas a last resort.

* **Fatigue.** Reporting of fatigue very common. Use of numbers effective to describe fatigue. Will take medications for fatigue or to sleep.

* **Depression.** Depression generally uncommon and patient may not recognize or report it.

* **Self-care for symptom management.** Avoid hospitals and doctors until illness is advanced. Very poor on long term care or medication. Tendency to stop self-care unless fearful of death or in great pain.

rth Rituals/Care of the New Mother/Baby

* **Pregnancy care.** Prenatal care generally avoided although more and more young Gypsies beginning to use it. Prefer not

to have internal examination and will avoid prenatal care to avoid such examinations. Need advice on healthy diet.

* **Labor practices.** Many deliveries performed by Gypsy midwife, but hospital deliveries increasingly accepted, usually on emergency basis when labor has begun. Offer pain relief though some may refuse it. Father usually not in room. Woman's mother may want to attend birth.

* **Role of the laboring woman during birth process.** Mother-to-be relies on assistance from older women relatives (mother, aunt, midwife). They inform her about what is happening only at time of labor, not before. Acceptance of modern birth practices increasing.

* **Role of the father and other family members during birth process.** Preferred coach is mother or aunt. Father stays outside birth room with other relatives. May absent himself altogether, not from lack of concern but from modesty at birth process.

* **Vaginal vs. cesarean section.** Vaginal delivery preferred. If cesarean section necessary, mother prefers to be conscious.

* **Breastfeeding.** Many young mothers do not breastfeed anymore, but in past breastfeeding was norm. Breastfeeding mothers avoid cabbage and other green vegetables and tomatoes, believing they give baby colic. Will drink beer or whiskey to calm baby.

* **Birth recuperation.** Women who have given birth are "polluted" (*mahrime*) for nine days because of birth fluids. Must not cook food or touch men. Hospital births popular because hospital disposes of birth fluids, thereby reducing woman's time in ritual pollution. Older women relatives may be near the new mother and baby but family members' visiting kept to minimum for fear of bringing in *Martiya*, spirit of night, who may harm baby.

* **Problems with baby.** If baby dies, parents must avoid it at all costs. May leave hospital suddenly. Grandparents responsible for burial of baby, but they too may leave everything to hospital to avoid bad luck of death.

    Babies often swaddled tightly. Believed to be very vulnerable to ev eye; visitors carefully watched lest t give baby evil eye. Fussing and/or colic viewed as evidence of evil eye. Giver of evil eye must make a cross with spittle on forehead of baby. If health care professional is asked to do so, best to comply. Nothing shameful about having evil eye as person cannot help it. People with bushy or heavy eyebrows or lots of body hair often have evil eye.

* **Male and female circumcision.** Male circumcision not traditionally done, but may be more acceptable due to more hospital births. Female circumcision unheard of.

Death Rituals

* **Preparation.** First inform eldest in authority and ask for help with relatives. Family may want priest present for purification of body. Family will want window open, preferably prior to death but also afterward, to allow spirit to leave.

  Grown children responsible for preparing funeral arrangements for parents. Subject of death avoided and may be discussed heatedly long before death. Dying person is anxious to have everything arranged for his/her death.

* **Home vs. hospital.** Preference varies by family, depending on illness and nature of death. For acute illness and those requiring extensive treatment, may prefer hospitalization. Critical issue is presence of family. For terminal stages of chronic illness, home stay most likely preferred.

* **Special needs.** May ask for religious object in room or favorite foods and personal article of dying person (such as his fishing pole). May even set up small home shrine. Will want to have older female relative at window at all times to keep out Night Spirits and chase them away and to allow dying person's spirit to be released. Moment of death highly significant. Feelings of dying person at that moment give relatives sense of what will happen in year after death. Last words very significant; close relatives will want to hear them.

* **Care of the body.** Body after death may be source of spiritual danger for relatives. Usually want it embalmed immediately to remove "blood." Will want to sit with body night and day after death where they can eat and drink. Funeral parlor usually most appropriate place.

Unless death very sudden, will have all
arrangements made.
* **Attitudes toward organ donation.** In past,
organ donation not accepted. Possible
but unlikely that attitudes have
changed recently.
* **Attitudes toward autopsy.** Very unlikely that
family would agree to autopsy. If medically necessary, eldest in authority
would decide.

Family Relationships
* **Composition/structure.** Composed of large
extended families of at least 3 generations, more often 4 to 5 generations.
Nuclear family size also large. Relatives
on both mother and father's side of
family important, but young person
resides and identifies usually with one
side of line (*vitsa*). Households include
3-4 generations and have fluid composition. All close relatives in town stay
at and eat at each other's houses.
Gather together daily, and relatives
from out-of-town visit constantly.
Family members fiercely loyal to each
other; therefore, when feuds break out
(usually between brothers vying for
authority), they cause irreparable splits
in family. Family takes strong interest
in arranging marriages of next generation. Remaining unmarried or being
gay or lesbian not acceptable option,
often leading to complete rejection
by community.
* **Decision making.** Individuals make their own
decisions, but prefer to consult entire
family first, and young people (35 and
under) often prefer to leave decisions
to older relatives. Eldest person usually
in authority. Men appear to be
spokesperson for whole family, but
older women (wife of spokesperson) a
critical part of decisions. She may in
fact have final word. Always consult
with both together to get lasting decision. Very old grandmother who is frail
may be past her time as authority figure, but if relatives defer to her, she
must be consulted too. Decisions
involving moral purity (*mahrime*) issues
may be out of immediate extended
family's hands and under jurisdiction of
all elders in area.
* **Spokesperson.** Parents speak for their children,
but also listen to wishes of child, often
to detriment of child's long term

health. Mother-in-law and father-in-law may make decisions for a daughter-in-law, but best to contact her parents.

* **Gender issues.** Men are ostensible leaders in political decision-making matters concerning group. Women play less obvious but crucial role. Women often principal money earners; men's work viewed as extra help. Men invest in women's careers. Women cook and care for children and are responsible for providing income for household (e.g., through fortune-telling). Men organize large festivities such as a *slava*, *pomana*, or baptism. Women generally keepers and communicators of medical and spiritual knowledge; thus their role very important in time of illness. Older women medical practitioners (*drabarnia*) may administer their own medicine in hospital in addition to medications ordered by doctor.

* **Caring role.** Women take primary role in caring for sick, but often do not follow instructions, instead providing their own notion of appropriate care. May have strong feelings about what patient needs and patient will accept decision, sometimes to his or her own detriment.

* **Expectations of and for children.** Children indulged and allowed to express themselves freely. Noisy, turbulent behavior tolerated though parents recognize that non-Gypsies have lower tolerance level. Children expected to grow up to be full members of group, that is, learn how to make a living in Gypsy way, marry person their parents approve of or select, have many children, and stay very close to families. Schooling not an expectation, but some children like to go for a few years; however, family activities take priority over schooling. Children expected to learn how to be savvy and street smart, how to talk their way out of situations, and to never accept anything at face value but to always check it out with other sources. Children learn at an early age to fend for themselves, to handle money correctly, and not to get cheated. Children very close to parents, siblings, and extended family members. Rebellion unusual but does occur.

* **Expectations of and for elders.** Elders highly respected for superior knowledge of

Gypsy culture and history, for long experience in dealing with non-Gypsies, and for ability to survive hardship. Elders also feared for their power to decide on membership in group or expulsion (worst punishment Gypsy can receive). Elders decide questions of moral purity and make all political decisions for group.

* **Expectations of adults in caring for children and elders.** Adults readily take on responsibilities of caring for children and elders without question. Have much help from many siblings, aunts, uncles, cousins, and in-laws. Gypsies will not go to nursing home or allow family member to go. Home care of elderly, sick, physically or mentally challenged, etc., always rests with family. Institutionalization of children or adults indicates that family is prepared to abandon individual completely; extremely rare event.

* **Expectation of visitors.** Large numbers of visitors a constant presence. If this presents difficulties, ask eldest in authority to organize system (e.g., five at a time) for room visits and to choose which close family members stay at all times (consult both male and female elder). Visitors to hospital can be managed by appealing to all elders to participate. Often works to designate room or area of garden where all Gypsies can gather. Outside is best, if weather permits. Gypsies prefer to segregate themselves from non-Gypsies and prefer to be outside where chances of being in contact with hospital *mahrime* (defined as lack of spiritual and moral cleanliness) are less. Designate one older person on hospital staff to manage large numbers of people and to answer questions and appeal to person(s) in authority to stay on top of situation and remain an effective liaison with hospital authorities.

Spiritual/Religious Orientation
* **Primary religious/spiritual affiliation.** Nominally Christian (Roman Catholic or Orthodox with some Pentecostal influence). Belief system related to spirits, saints, and other supernatural beings motivates death rituals and Saint's Day celebrations. Shrine in home is common.

* **Usual religious/spiritual practices.** Family may bring in figures of saints and other objects of spiritual importance.
* **Use of spiritual healing/healers.** Family may ask for presence of priest or chaplain. Older female relative who is also spiritual healer (*drabarni*) may bring in certain plants and medicines to give patient.

Illness Beliefs

* **Causes of physical illness.** Health, good luck, and prosperity all result of spiritual and moral cleanliness (*wuzho*). Lack of spiritual and moral cleanliness (*mahrime*) not only results in disease and bad luck, but attracts certain spirits (*mamioro, Martiya*) or devil (*o beng*), harbingers of illness.
* **Causes of mental illness.** Extremely rare, but mental illness is defined generally as non-conformist (to Gypsy culture) behavior. Cure is to conform. Gypsy who does not want to marry, which is sign of mental illness, for example, is cured by marrying.
* **Causes of genetic defects.** Gypsies accepting of genetic, birth, or congenital defects, do not distinguish significantly among them, and take care of their loved ones at home. Generally will refuse institutionalization.
* **Sick role.** Sick persons expect family to attend to needs and care for them. Since illness is a group crisis as well as an individual one, patient must deal with both aspects of disease.
* **Home and folk remedies.** Devil causes convulsions (cured by giving patient feces of devil, thought to be *asafetida*) and *Mamioro* brings a number of serious illnesses such as flu, pneumonia, TB, cholera, and plague (cured by giving patient *Mamioro's* vomit, thought to be slime mold, (*Fuligo septica*). Regardless of these beliefs, Gypsies are imminently practical and recognize that "American doctors" are also powerful healers and have very effective medicine. Frequently use both just to make sure patient recovers.
* **Acceptance of procedures.** Invasive procedures and operations ("going under the knife") highly feared. Use of anesthesia also feared and viewed as "little death." Both should be very carefully

explained to minimize fear and emphasize benefits to patient. If operation
not perceived as life and death issue,
many Gypsies will refuse it.
Gynecologic or proctologic exams
highly embarrassing and shocking.
Perform only when absolutely
necessary and when necessity has
been fully explained.

*   **Care seeking.** Gypsies use own medicines,
    based on their own theories of causes
    of illness, concurrently with
    "American medicine," based on germ
    theory, for example.

Health Practices

*   **Concept of health.** Good health related to
    moral purity, keeping upper and lower
    halves of body separate, and good
    behavior. Good health, prosperity,
    large families, and good luck inextrica-
    bly intertwined. Knowledge of anato-
    my extremely weak.
*   **Health promotion and prevention.**
    Promotion of good health means
    staying clean (*wuzho*) and avoiding
    unclean (*mahrime*). Very little knowl-
    edge of preventive medicine, healthy
    eating practices, or exercise. Often
    heavy smokers and drinkers.
*   **Screening.** Important to explain reasons for
    screening in relation to notion of
    health in general. Screening for
    sexually transmitted diseases likely
    to be resisted.

Selected References

Bodner, A., & Leininger, M. (1992). Transcultural
nursing care values, beliefs, and practices of American
(USA) Gypsies. *Journal of Transcultural Nursing, 4*(1),
17-28.

Sutherland, A. (1992). Health and illness among the
Rom of California. *Journal of the Gypsy Lore Society,*
5(2), No.1., 19-59.

Sutherland, A. (1992). Gypsies and health care. *Western
Journal of Medicine, 157*(3), 276-280.

Thomas, J. (1987). Disease, lifestyle, and consanguinity
in 58 American Gypsies. *Lancet, 2*, 377-379.

Author

Anne H. Sutherland, DPhil is Professor of
Anthropology at Macalester College, St. Paul,

Minnesota and has studied *Roma* Gypsies in the U.S. for 28 years. She is the author of *Gypsies, the Hidden Americans* (Waveland Press, 1986) and numerous articles on the medical and legal system of Gypsies.

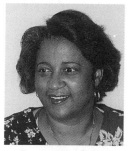

Jessie M. Colin

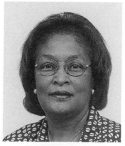

Ghislaine
Paperwalla

Cultural/Ethnic Identity

* **Preferred terms**. No particular preferred
    terms other than Haitian or
    Haitian-American.

* **History of immigration/migration.**

    Before 1920, Haitians traveled only for
    educational purposes. They learned a
    profession and returned to Haiti to put
    it into practice.

1920   First significant group of Haitian
                immigrants migrated to U.S.
                because of atrocities that accom-
                panied American occupation of
                Haiti during 1915-1934. This first
                group of Haitians is believed to
                have settled in Harlem and assimi-
                lated into American society.

1957   Francois Duvalier became presi-
                dent of Haiti. This period started
                the "real" migration of Haitians.
                Those who left were politicians
                whose aim was to organize and
                overthrow Duvalier's regime.

                Educated professionals also
                left Haiti in search of a better life.
                They were able to settle and
                quickly send for their families.

1964   Duvalier was elected president for
                life. This led to a significant num-
                ber of Haitians fleeing the island,
                primarily relatives of politicians
                who opposed the Duvalier regime.
                The majority of those who had
                migrated up to this time had legal-
                ly entered U.S.

1971   Francois Duvalier died and was
                succeeded by his son Jean-Claude,
                also appointed for life at age 19.
                Haiti was also suffering from eco-
                nomic deprivation, motivating
                another major exodus of immi-
                grants consisting of urbanites and
                peasants. Many were unable to pay

for their transportation, passports,
and American visas, and started
coming to the country covertly on
small sailboats.

1980-present Immigration branched into
two groups: those who came legally and those who entered the
U.S. through the underground.
This latter group came via high
seas and thus were called "boat
people."

* **Map page.** *See Appendix C, p. 2.*

Communication

* **Major language(s) and dialects.** Two official
languages in Haiti: French and Creole,
designated by 1987 Haitian constitu-
tion. Creole is the national language
spoken by entire population of Haiti,
and the language used by people of
Haitian descent born or living abroad.

  Haiti has an oral culture, with a
long tradition of proverbs, jokes, and
stories reflecting on philosophical systems. These are used as educational
tools to pass on unwritten knowledge.
These jokes and proverbs are also used
to communicate emotions and convey
messages, i.e.,
Pale franse pa di lespri pou sa (To speak
French doesn't mean you are smart);
Kreyol pale, Kreyol kompran (What you
hear is what I say).

* **Literacy assessment.** Haiti is a non-literate
culture. Eighty percent or more of
people neither read nor write. Thus
educational material about health
should be visual and oral (i.e., video,
radio programs).

* **Nonverbal communication.** Affectionate,
polite, but shy. Uneducated Haitians
generally do not show their lack of
knowledge to non-Haitians, but keep
to themselves and avoid conflict,
sometimes projecting a timid attitude.
More comfortable with non-English
speaking immigrants, especially
islanders, because they feel a common
bond. While interacting with an
American, if they don't understand,
they will still show approval by nodding rather than expose their limitations. They smile a lot and avoid eye
contact as much as possible, especially
with those in position of authority.

* **Use of interpreters.** Interpreters mistrusted
because of belief that they generally do

not accurately convey the intended message. Prefer to use family members rather than friends because they are very keen on maintaining confidentiality. Without a family member, would rather use professional interpreter with whom they have no relationship and will likely never see again.

* **Greetings.** Very friendly: embrace and kiss as sign of affection and acceptance in informal situations. In formal encounters, shake hands as sign of greeting, are composed and stern in formal situations.

  Gender also plays significant role in formal situation. For example, a man will not embrace a woman in a formal setting, even if they are friends. The polite and respectful salutation is a handshake.

* **Tone of voice.** Haitian language very rich and expressive. Voice intonation conveys emotions. Pitch is high or low, depending on the message. Tone expresses joy or sadness, happiness or deceit. Haitians are very expressive and tend to get loud, generally accompanied by hand gestures as a means of reinforcement or emphasis, especially when discussing issues of particular interest (e.g., politics).

* **Orientation toward time.** Not committed to time or schedule; perception of time is unrealistic. Not impolite to arrive late for an appointment; everyone and anything can wait. In fact, Haitians compensate by manipulating timing of activities. For example, a wedding invitation will show a starting time of 6 pm, when the actual starting time is in fact 7 or 7:30 pm. This practice pervades Haitian society. They may be timely for medical appointments if being on time was emphasized when the appointment was made.

* **Consents.** Generally give impression that they do not want to know and do not want informed consent.

  Haitians are trusting of expert, believing that expert has their interest at heart and is more knowledgeable than they. Therefore, the expert has authority to dictate what should be done. To obtain consent, it is important to indicate clearly importance of procedure and absolute need for consent. Ask a family member whom the patient chooses to be present through-out the interaction.

* **Privacy.** Haitians are very private, only reveal-ing what is of utmost necessity. Will not disclose information even if neces-sary if they are not ready for that dis-closure. Shame concept is real: their body is not to be exposed. Private even with themselves: for example, women should not touch their own bodies. As a result, teaching breast self-examination is very difficult because it teaches something they have been programmed not to do.

    Will not appreciate a health care worker talking about their condition with a friend or family member if they have not given permission. Will not outwardly express their disapproval; however, relationship with health care worker will be automatically severed. The nurse or health care worker will not even realize the breakdown in rela-tionship until it's too late.

* **Serious or terminal illness.** There are varying degrees of illnesses. Serious or terminal illnesses are expressed in the following ways:
    Moin malad anpil (I am very sick) means the person is in critical condition.
    Moin pap refe (I will never be well again) means that the client is termi-nal and that death is imminent. Haitians have a fatalistic view about illness, reflected in the following expression which shows optimism and fatalism:
    Bondye, Bon (God is good) Whatever happens is God's will, and what God does is for the best.

    When dealing with terminal illness, first inform closest member of family or person in charge. That per-son will find ways of informing the patient if they think it necessary. Same procedure should be followed in case of surgery, especially abdominal surgery, since this type of surgery is generally feared.

Activities of Daily Living

* **Modesty.** Both men and women very modest. Men embarrassed by hospital gowns, so offer hospital pajamas. If planned hospital stay, patients bring own gown or pajamas.

Gender plays an important role in health care interactions: physicians should be male, nurses should be female. To Haitians, both these groups are highly respected and trusted.

* **Skin care.** Shower daily, preferably in the morning. Women perform thorough peri-care with soap at night before bedtime. Lotion used mostly by more educated Haitians.

* **Hair care.** Women shampoo weekly, use rollers at night to maintain style. Oil based pomades used to replenish the scalp and to keep hair from drying. Men shampoo daily with shower.

* **Nail care.** Less educated Haitian women keep nails short and devoid of all polish. Those more educated will have manicures and pedicures weekly.

* **Toileting.** Because they are very private, will insist on using the bathroom. If family member can assist, patient may use bedpan or urinal. Perianal care is performed after using the toilet. This means pouring water over the perineal area and the anus, soaping, washing, and drying thoroughly.

* **Special clothing or amulets.** Haitians predominantly Catholic, will often have religious medallions, rosary beads, or figure of a saint to whom they are devoted.

    Voodooism is an important religious component, an African spirit religion closely related to Catholicism. Saints worshiped by Catholic Church are same as used in *voodooism*, but with different names and functions. Therefore, picture of a saint in patient room may have double meaning, but generally there for protection. Do not remove anything of this kind from patient's room unless interfering with care. If it must be removed, be sure to seek permission.

* **Self-care.** During initial stages of illness, family will want to help with patient's hygiene, again related to privacy issue. They will wait for specific direction on what to do in performing care. Therefore, it is important to be specific about what patient or family can do for themselves. Offer assistance whenever possible; remember, they want to be clean, feel clean, and smell clean.

    Because of fear of surgery (especially abdominal), patients will limit self-care activities, believing that any physical strain may have a negative effect on the body. Need to be strongly encouraged to cough, deep breathe, and ambulate to avoid complications.

Food Practices

* **Usual meal pattern.** Generally eat largest meal at lunch time. Breakfast generally consists of bread, butter and coffee, and dinner is soup or hot cereal. In U.S., some have adjusted to routines here, for example, eating their heaviest meal at dinner.

* **Food beliefs and rituals.** Hot/cold disequilibrium. Illness also believed to be caused when the body is exposed to an imbalance of "cold" (*fret*) and "hot" (*cho*) factors. For example, eating tomatoes or white beans after childbirth believed to induce hemorrhage, and cold orange juice avoided during menstruation. Food also considered in terms of heavy or light qualities: heavy foods such as cornmeal mush, broiled plantain, or potato should be eaten during the day to provide energy for the workday. Light foods such as hot chocolate milk, bread, or soup usually eaten for dinner because easily digestible. Method of preparation also considered; boiled green plantains are heavy but fried yellow/ripped plantain considered light.

* **Usual diet.** Haitians not explorers when it comes to food. In hospital, prefer fasting to eating non-Haitian food, afraid that such food may make them more sick. Types of food preferred are rice, beans, plantain, spicy braised meat with gravy or stewed vegetables, and chicken.

  Haitians do not eat yogurt, cottage cheese, or runny egg yolk. Prefer rolls and French bread rather than sliced bread.

* **Fluids.** Drink a lot of water and homemade fruit juices, cold fruity soda, coffee in the morning, tea only when sick.

* **Food prohibitions.** Food prohibitions related to particular diseases and particular stages of life cycle. For example, teenagers advised to refrain from drinking citrus juices such as orange or lemon, to avoid development of acne.

  After performing strenuous activity, or any activity which causes body to become hot, one should not eat cold food since that will throw the body into a state of *chofret* (i.e., pineapple is cold food; if eaten after excessive walking, pineapple could cause gastric hemorrhage).

* **Food prescriptions.** During illness, Haitians like pumpkin soup, bouillon, special soup made with green vegetable, meat, plantain, dumplings, and yam. Also like all kinds of porridge, oatmeal, cream of corn meal prepared with milk, sugar, cinnamon, vanilla flavoring, and pinch of salt (called *Akasan*).

Symptom Management

* **Pain.** Commonly referred to as *doule*. Haitians have very low pain threshold. Whole demeanor changes, very verbal about what is paining them, sometimes moaning. Usually very vague about location of pain, believing that whole body system affected; therefore, location of pain is not important since disease travels. Injection the preferred treatment method, followed by elixir, tablets, and finally, capsules.

  Chest pain referred to as *doule nan ke mwen*, abdominal pain is *doule nan vent*, stomach pain is also referred to as *doule nan ke mwen* or *doule nan lestomak mwen*.

* **Dyspnea.** A primary respiratory ailment is *oppression*, a term used to describe asthma, but includes more than asthma. Seems to describe a state of anxiety and hyperventilation instead of asthma. *Oppression* considered a "cold" state, as are many respiratory conditions. Patient will say *M ap toufe* or *mwen pa ka respire*.

  Oxygen should be offered only when absolutely necessary since use of oxygen is associated with seriousness of disease.

* **Nausea/Vomiting.** Nausea is expressed as *lestomak-mwen ap roule*, *M santi m anvi vomi*, *lestomak-mwen chaje*, or *ke mwen tounin*. Those more educated will express their discomfort as nausea. Because of modesty, they will dispense of any vomitus immediately so as not to upset others. Specific instructions should be given regarding keeping the specimen.

* **Constipation/Diarrhea.** Referred to as *konstipasyon*, treated with laxative or some herbal tea. Sometimes will use enemas (*lavman*).

  Diarrhea not a major concern in adults; however, considered very dangerous in children and sometimes interpreted as a hex on the child. Will try herbal medicine, seek help from a voodoo priest (*hougan*), and, if all else fails, may use a physician. Very important to assess child carefully because he may have been ill for quite some time.

* **Fatigue.** Seen as sign of physical weakness known as *febles*, and interpreted as sign of anemia, or insufficient blood. Symptoms generally attributed to poor diet. Patient may suggest to health professional a need for special care, meaning to eat well, take vitamins, and rest. Will eat liver, pigeon meat, watercress, bouillon made of green leafy vegetables, cow's feet, and red meat to counteract the *febles*.

* **Depression.** Haitians in U.S. strongly resist acculturation, taking pride in preserving traditional spiritual, religious, and family values. Stigma against mental illness is so strong that Haitians will not readily admit to depression. Major factor to keep in mind is strong prevalence of voodoo which deals with depression as possession by malevolent spirits or punishment for not honoring good protective spirits. Depression can also be viewed as hex put on by a jealous or envious individual.

  Factors that may trigger depression are memories of family in homeland, thinking about spirits in Haiti, dreams about dead family, guilt and regrets about abandoning family in Haiti for abundance in the U.S.

  Need to be sensitive to root cause of problem, ascertain need for comfort within particular religious beliefs.

* **Self-care for symptom management.** Haitian try home remedies as first resort for treating illness. They are self-diagnosticians with home remedies for a particular ailment or, if they know someone who had a particular illness, they may take the prescribed medicine from that person.

  A patient may use another Haitian's experience with a particular illness as a barometer on which to measure their symptoms and institute treatment. If necessary, a person living in the U.S. may ask friends or relatives to send medications from Haiti. Such medications may consist of roots, leaves, and European manufactured products that are more familiar.

Another condition which should be assessed is fright or *sezisman*. Various external and internal environmental factors are believed to cause sezisman, thereby throwing the normal blood into disruption. *Sezisman* may occur when someone receives bad news or is involved in a frightful situation, or suffers from indignation after being unjustly treated. When this condition occurs, blood is said to move to the head, causing partial loss of vision, headache, increased blood pressure, and/or a stroke. To counteract this occurrence, patient may sit quietly, put a cold compress on the forehead, drink bitter herbal tea, or take sips of water.

Birth Rituals/Care of the New Mother/Baby

* **Pregnancy care.** Pregnancy care is not seen as a health problem but a happy time for entire family. Pregnancy does not relieve the women from her work; she is expected to fulfill her obligation throughout pregnancy.

    Pregnant women experience an increase in salivation, and Haitian women rid themselves of the excess at places that may seem inappropriate. Sometimes they carry a "spit" cup with them and are not embarrassed by this behavior. They do not believe that they should swallow their saliva. Others need to be tolerant of this behavior since excess salivation is a natural effect of pregnancy.

    Pregnant women are restricted from eating spices because they may irritate the child. However, they are permitted to eat vegetables and red fruits, believing that this will build up the child's blood. Encouraged to eat a lot because they are eating for two.

    Some may seek prenatal care at private physician's office or at a clinic. Generally, however, many Haitian women do not seek prenatal care.

* **Labor practices.** May walk, pace, sit, squat, and rub her belly; will not ask for analgesics.

* **Role of the laboring woman during birth process.** Plays an active role during this process: talks loud, may scream, curse and sometimes even becomes hysterical. Some are stoic, only moaning or grunting.

* **Role of the father and other family members during birth process.** Father a non-participant, remaining outside of the process. Believes this a private event best handled by women. Woman not coached; however, female family members will give assistance as needed if midwife involved.

* **Vaginal vs. cesarean section.** Vaginal delivery more common, natural child-birth the norm. Women in higher social strata quicker to have cesarean. C-section feared, however, because abdominal surgery.

* **Breastfeeding.** Encouraged for up to 9 months postpartum. Milk of lactating woman believed to be stored in her breast, and can become detrimental to both mother and child if it becomes too thick or too thin. If too thin, it is believed that milk has "turned" and may cause diarrhea in the child, headache and possible postpartum depression in the mother. If milk is too thick, may cause impetigo (*bouton*). Mixed feedings (breast and bottle) very much accepted. If child develops diarrhea, breastfeeding immediately discontinued.

* **Birth recuperation.** Very important period for Haitian woman. Takes an active role in own care, dresses warmly, takes baths (*vapors*), and drinks tea, in order to be rejuvenated. Belief that first three days postpartum should be on bed rest, avoid drafts, and not venture out during the night. One major practice is that of the three baths: special leaves are gathered and boiled to make a special water for hot bathing during the first three days postpartum, and the woman is encouraged to drink tea boiled from these same leaves. For the next three days, the mother bathes in a special water in which leaves have been soaked and warmed by the sun. About 1 month postpartum, the mother takes the third bath, a cold bath. The third bath enhances healing, tightens muscles and bones which been loosened during delivery.

After childbirth, woman believed to be particularly susceptible to entry of gas (*gaz*) into the body. To prevent this, she must tighten her waist with a piece of linen or a belt. Procedure also important to tighten woman's bones loosened by birth of her child.

Food restrictions important in this phase and include not eating white food (i.e., milk, white lima beans, lobster, tomatoes, etc.), considered cold food. Eating cold food believed to increase vaginal discharge and/or hemorrhage. Acceptable foods include cornmeal mush or porridge, red bean sauce, rice and beans, and plantain.

* **Problems with baby.** Maternal grandmother first person summoned if problems with child. Home remedies tried first.
* **Male and female circumcision.** Females not circumcised. Male circumcision not encouraged. Believed that male circumcision decreases sexual satisfaction.

Death Rituals

* **Preparation.** Death mobilizes entire extended family. Death arrangements usually taken care of by elder kinsman of dying. Kinsman generally responsible to notify all family members wherever they may be; their travel plans will influence funeral arrangements. Kinsman also makes arrangements for burial services, for pre-burial activities (called *veye*), orders coffin, makes arrangement for prayer services before the funeral, and makes contact regarding the funeral services.

  Dernie priye is a special prayer service consisting of seven consecutive days of prayer. Usually takes place in the home. Purpose is to facilitate passage of the soul from this world to the next. On the seventh day, there is a mass called *prise de deuil*, which begins the official mourning process. Each of these activities concludes with a reception/celebration in memory of the departed.

  Cremation not acceptable option because of deep respect for the body and the belief in resurrection and paradise.

* **Home vs. hospital.** Haitians prefer to be at home. However, since migrating to U.S., they have accepted death at the hospital because of heavy burden on

the family during terminal illness.
Generally, however, Haitians prefer to
be cared for at home.

* **Special needs.** When death is imminent, family will pray, cry uncontrollably, even hysterically. They try to meet spiritual needs of dying person by bringing religious medallions, pictures of saints, or fetish. Because of their deep respect for the dead, the body is kept until all family members can be present for the service.

* **Care of the body.** Final bath given by a family member. If not too disturbing for the nursing unit, allow family to participate in postmortem care.

* **Attitudes toward organ donation.** Neither dealt with nor encouraged.

* **Attitudes toward autopsy.** Haitians very cautious about this procedure. However, if foul play or unnatural death suspected, will request an autopsy to ensure that the patient is really dead. The practice of zombification (the creation of zombies occurs due to malice or greed) is prevalent more with rural community than urban areas. Zombies are people who respond to commands and have no "free will."

Family Relationships

* **Composition/structure.** Close, tightly knit extended family and nuclear family. Sometimes large family group lives together under one roof and in small quarters. Gay and lesbian relationships are not acknowledged.

* **Decision making.** Matriarchal society, but men are allowed to believe they are head of household. Man relinquishes all responsibilities to mate, especially those involved with management of household and care of children.

* **Spokesperson.** Depending on situation, may be father or mother or elder kinsman/person in position of authority in that family unit.

* **Gender issues.** Haitian society projects image of chauvinism. However, women really backbone of family unit.

* **Caring role.** Generally, women assume caring responsibilities. Men supposed to project image of strength and not display emotion.

* **Expectations of and for children.** Children expected to be respectful, caring, and obedient. Cared for by both parents in

highly protective, secure environment. Expected to be high achievers, especially in educational domain. There is a proverb that says *sa ki lan men ou se li ki pa ou*, meaning "what's in your hand is what you have;" education can never be taken away from you.

* **Expectations of and for elders.** Elders highly respected. Children expected to care for and provide for them. Elders are the family advisors, baby sitters, historians, and consultants.

* **Expectations of adults in caring for children and elders.** Children sent to boarding school to pursue education. Elderly usually cared for at home. Migration to U.S. poses tremendous challenges, that is, caring for elders while working outside the home. Small percentage deciding reluctantly to place elders in nursing homes.

* **Expectation of visitors.** Visits from close friends or family encouraged. Friends or family help maintain comfort of patient around the clock until they feel that patient ready to be independent.

Spiritual/Religious Orientation

* **Primary religious/spiritual affiliation.** Primary religious affiliation is Catholicism. Since 1970s, Protestantism has mushroomed. Believed that about 15-20% of Haitians are Protestant.

    Voodooism another major religion in Haiti. Taken very seriously and not only by peasants and unlettered.

* **Usual religious/spiritual practices.** Receive holy communion often. Pray using rosary beads, practice novenas; may select a saint to pray to, wear only colors associated with that saint for a predetermined time period. Believe in power of prayers for physical healing.

    Strongly believe in all sacraments; very fearful of Sacrament of the Sick which they equate with death.

* **Use of spiritual healing/healers.** Voodoo priest (*mambo* or *hougan*) definitely sought by believers who need to worship the spirit to be relieved of illness.

Illness Beliefs

* **Causes of physical illness.** Physical illness thought to be on a continuum

beginning with *Kom pa bon*, (I do not feel well). The affected person is not confined to bed; illness is transitory, and the person should soon be able to return to their normal activities. The next phase is *moin malad* (I am sick). A third phase is *moin malad anpil*, (I am very sick). This means the person is very ill. The final phase is *Moin pap refe*, (I am dying).

Illness perceived as punishment, considered an assault on the body and may have two different etiologies:

Natural illness, known as *maladi bon die* (disease of the Lord), illness of short duration. May occur frequently and is caused by environmental factors such as food, air, cold, heat, and gas. Other causes of natural illness are movement of blood within the body, disequilibrium between hot and cold, and bone displacement.

Supernatural illness, on the other hand, is very serious, and attributed to spirits' (*loa*) anger. This happens when the body that the *loa* inhabits deceives it.

* **Causes of mental illness.** Mental illness is not well accepted and usually believed to have supernatural causes.
* **Causes of genetic defects.** Physical deformity brought on by an angry spirit perhaps enlisted by an enemy.
* **Sick role.** Sick person assumes a passive role and allows others to do for him. Family members will rise to the occasion with everyone participating in the care of the loved one.
* **Home and folk remedies.** Usually the first line of treatment, and may include tea, massage, *benye fey cho* (hot bath with boiled leaves), poultice.
* **Acceptance of procedures.** Procedure should be explained clearly and slowly. Use of a trusted interpreter essential.
* **Care seeking.** Very strong belief in God's power and ability to heal. God's work done through various media, including dreams, traditional and medical means. Seek medical care when established that illness requires medical attention.

Health Practices
* **Concept of health.** Good health seen as the maintenance of equilibrium. To achieve this state, one must eat well, give attention to personal hygiene.

Prayer and good spiritual habits very important to achieve healthy balance.

* **Health promotion and prevention.** To promote health, one must be strong, have good color, be plump, and have no pain. To maintain this state, one must eat right, sleep right, keep warm, exercise, and keep clean. The most important exercise for Haitians is walking, which is so ingrained into day-to-day activity that it is not seen as exercise.

  Haitians engage in self treatment activities and see it as ways of promoting health or preventing disease (i.e., the person who suspects a venereal disease may buy penicillin and have someone administer it; for a minor cold, may take antibiotics given by a friend).

  In the summer, Haitian parents engage their children in certain health promotion activities such as giving them *lok*, a mixture of bitter tea leaves, juice, sugar cane syrup, and oil. In addition, children are also given *lavman* (enemas) to ensure cleanliness. This is also supposed to rid the bowel of impurities and refresh it, prevent acne, and rejuvenate the body.

* **Screening**. Screening a well accepted concept although Haitians will not admit to diseases, especially contagious diseases. Very respectful of doctors and nurses. Physicians are male; nurses are female, referred to as "Miss."

Selected References

Desantis, L., & Thomas, J. (1992). Health education and the immigrant mother: Cultural insights for community health nurses. *Public Health Nursing, 9*(2), 87-96.

Harris, K. (1987). Beliefs and practices among Haitian Americans in relation to child bearing. *Journal of Nurse-Midwifery, 32*(3), 149-155.

Laguerre, M. S. (1981). Haitian Americans. In A. Harwood (Ed.), *Ethnicity and medical care* (pp. 172-210). Cambridge: Harvard University Press.

Laguerre, M.S. (1984). *American odyssey: Haitians in New York City*. Ithaca: Cornell University Press.

Rasanbleman, F. A. (1976). *Congres Mondiale pour L'annee Internationale de la Femme* (pp 1-58). Montreal: Canada.

Authors

Jessie M. Colin, RN, MSN is Assistant Professor of Nursing at Barry University in Miami Shores, Florida. She is a doctoral student at Adelphi University, New York and is interested in studying the meaning of Haitian adolescents living in another culture. She is Haitian-American and migrated to the U.S. as an adolescent. She was co-Founder of the Haitian Health Foundation of South Florida and a member of the Haitian American Nurses Association of Florida.

Ghislaine Paperwalla, RN, BSN is a Research Nurse in Immunology at the Veterans Administration Medical Center in Miami, Florida. Born in Haiti and immigrated to the U.S. in 1960, she received her nursing education at Laval University in Canada and Florida International University. She is President of the Haitian American Nurses Association of Florida and Vice President of the Haitian Health Foundation of South Florida.

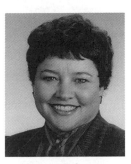

Sharon Johnson

Cultural/Ethnic Identity

* **Preferred term.** Hmong, which means human being in Hmong language.
* **History of immigration**. Immigration began in 1975 after Vietnam War. New immigrants have continued to enter U.S. as late as 1995, sponsored by family members who immigrated earlier.

     Hmong people found in Southeast Asian areas of southern China, Laos, Vietnam, Burma, and Thailand. Thought to be indigenous people of Yellow River area of China. Tend to live in high mountainous areas in Southeast Asia. Because of geographical isolation, have retained own unique language and customs. Life in homeland rugged: no running water or electricity. Life expectancy short.

     The Hmong in U.S. are originally from Laos but may have lived many years in Thailand refugee camps. During Vietnam War, fought for U.S. Central Intelligence Agency against Communists. When war ended, they were targeted for genocide by Communists who controlled Laos. Many Hmong were killed or injured in military onslaughts and biological/chemical warfare.

     After immigration to U.S., a second migration occurred in which families and clans were reunited. Migration continues as Hmong families move to areas of U.S. with employment opportunities.
* **Map page.** *See Appendix C, p. 6.*

Communication

* **Major language(s) and dialects.** Most older people speak only Hmong although men may also speak Lao since many served in Laos military or worked for

Laos government. There are two
Hmong dialects, White and Green
(sometimes called Blue). Younger
people tend to be bilingual, speaking
both English and Hmong, although
many have only rudimentary Hmong
language skills and are not adequate
interpreters for medicolegal situations.

* **Literacy assessment.** Written Hmong language
not developed until 1950s. Most older
Hmong have no formal schooling and
are not literate in their own language
or in English. Young people will be literate in English but may not be able to
read Hmong or Lao although there is
an effort in Hmong community to
teach young people to speak and read
their traditional language.

* **Nonverbal communication.** Hmong people
very polite and reticent. Very aware of
disrespectful and prejudicial behavior,
but will not protest to health care professional. Consider prolonged, direct
eye contact rude. Physical affection
and touching not done in public but
health care professional's touching may
be accepted as "the way Americans
are." Tend to communicate indirectly
and try to present positive image.
Many will not say "no" outright but
will say "I'll think about it" when they
don't wish to do something. "Yes" can
mean "yes," but may also mean "I hear
you;" it does not necessarily mean
affirmative response.

* **Use of interpreters.** Many Hmong will want
their own trusted relatives who are
bilingual to be present. Hmong interpreters employed by hospital or institution considered loyal to hospital and
may be distrusted. Children rarely
good interpreters because they lack
adequate Hmong language skills. For
many families, however, young bilingual adults most likely working and it
may be difficult or impossible for them
to bring in an adult interpreter.
Hmong men and women may not discuss or admit to intimate problems to
an interpreter of opposite sex.

Hmong language structure considerably different from Indo-European
languages. When working with interpreters, important to give entire sentence, paragraph, or thought, so they
know intent of message necessary for
accurate interpretation. Hmong

language lacks many terms comparable to English and has almost no medical terms. Procedures may be interpreted in most rudimentary way and/or erroneously.

Hmong people have great respect for authority and "saving face" is important. Interpreter may not understand what you have said but may not tell you. Ensuring that interpreter understands your questions is first step to accurate communication with patient. Interpreter may not want to interpret comments considered rude in Hmong culture.

Also, interpreter of one sex may feel it is not proper to discuss some topics with patient of opposite sex. Before interpreting takes place, talk with interpreter to assess the level of comfort with the planned questions and discussion.

* **Greetings.** Handshakes, smiles, and introductions appropriate. Most older Hmong women usually retain their own surname after marriage. Younger women may have adopted husband's surname. Do not refer to Hmong patients by their first names; use Mr. or Mrs. and last name. Calling married woman by first name considered inappropriate and disrespectful to her husband.

* **Tone of voice.** Tone of voice should be modulated.

* **Orientation toward time.** Many older Hmong individuals are present-oriented. Calendars and clocks rarely used in rural Laos and many Hmong born in Laos do not know their actual birthdates. Many birthdates assigned in refugee camps, resulting in some erroneous ages, so people may actually be younger or older than their stated age.

Keeping appointment times has been difficult. Hmong patients may arrive early in morning on day of their medical appointment. This occurs less often as children serve as socializers to Western system. Social events within Hmong community may start several hours after stated time.

* **Consents.** Many Hmong people suspicious of consent forms if they cannot read them and are afraid that form does not contain what was explained orally. Rumors persist in Hmong community that American doctors "practice" on

Hmong people because Hmong are uneducated about Western medical system. May be suspicious of health care professional's motives, especially if care provided by students.

Surgery rarely available to Hmong in Laos so they are especially afraid of surgical procedures. Patient will often want family members (usually male elders) to review consent forms before signing. This can lead to considerable delays before treatment can begin since elders may not be readily available. Lack of elder availability may also be used as delaying tactic when family either needs more time to make decision or does not want procedure or surgery, yet does not want to directly state their decision (See Communication).

* **Privacy.** Hmong families tend to be large, and privacy within family often lacking. Many will not feel comfortable sleeping in hospital alone, but will want another family member with them at all times. Hmong folktales warn that evil befalls Hmong person who goes out alone.

Adult women are modest and will not feel comfortable having a physical examination. Purpose of examination must be clearly explained before consent can be obtained. Women often will refuse pelvic examinations by male health care providers but will more likely accept them from female practitioner.

Concerns of a private nature may not be freely revealed unless asked directly. If interpreter of opposite sex, patient may deny that problem exists. However, males are especially sensitive to topics such as impotence and will deny this problem even in presence of male Hmong interpreter. Sensitive information can sometimes be obtained if question first presented with explanation that "this is a common problem for all people who have your diagnosis, and I am wondering if this might be a concern of yours also?"

* **Serious or terminal illness.** Hmong people present positive attitude in presence of seriously ill family members. May visit someone they know is dying and say that they're sure the patient will "get well soon." Considered inappropriate

to speak of impending death to someone with fatal diagnosis. This may be due to traditional belief that evil spirit may be cause of illness and if complications or potentially fatal outcomes spoken about in front of patient, evil spirit will then know what to do.

This cultural perspective problematic in Western medical system where Patient's Bill of Rights states that patient has right to knowledge regarding his or her diagnosis. Hmong people may be so shocked by abruptly presented information that they may leave and never return. Better to discuss sensitive issues with family first and ask them how best to convey this information to patient.

Activities of Daily Living

* **Modesty.** Hmong women's perspectives regarding their bodies can vary considerably. Older women modest regarding their genitals but because of past breastfeeding experiences, may not be concerned about baring their breasts. Some older women may forget to button their blouses and not be concerned about exposure. Men are modest but accept examination of their genitals by female health care professionals as appropriate to their problems.

* **Skin care.** Bathing infrequent in Laos due to water being available only from well or stream. In U.S., daily bathing more commonly expected.

* **Hair care.** Women do not shampoo daily if hair very long (common in this culture).

* **Nail care.** No known restrictions.

* **Toileting.** No known restrictions or concerns.

* **Special clothing/amulets.** Traditional Hmong people may wear amulets at neck, wrists, waist, and/or ankles. These may be gold necklaces or bracelets, string, fabric bands, or chains. Small amulet pouches may be attached. These thought to have special powers to hold the soul in and keep evil spirits out, and should not be removed without permission.

If Hmong person has had shaman ritual to treat illness, blood of sacrificed animal may be placed on clothing. Parts of animal (such as nails or teeth) may be placed in pocket on their back or sewn onto clothing.

May not want this clothing removed since its purpose is to have spirit of dead animal protect ill person. (Note: Christian Hmong do not practice shaman healing rituals.)

* **Self-care.** When ill, Hmong person expects female family members to provide care. Women primary caregivers, and daughters-in-law are expected to provide care for in-laws.

Food Practices

* **Usual meal pattern.** Hmong usually eat two to three meals a day. If person customarily eats two meals per day, first meal is usually about 9 or 10 am and second in late afternoon or early evening. Same types of foods eaten at each meal.

* **Food beliefs and rituals.** Hmong people eat special foods when ill or not feeling well, such as plain boiled rice soup which may contain small amounts of chicken. Hmong suspicious of store-bought chicken and meat, believing these contain unhealthful chemicals. Many prefer to kill their own live chickens and animals or to purchase meat fresh. Appearance of chicken (e.g., color of chicken feet) enters into their beliefs regarding benefit of that chicken as healing food.

* **Usual diet.** Rice main staple along with small amounts of meat, fish, and green vegetables. Noodle dishes and soups also favorites. Large amounts of MSG often used by some people. Food usually bland but hot chili condiments and salty sauces may be added at table to individual taste. Fruit rarely eaten. Sweets and soda adopted as American favorites.

* **Fluids.** Women have special prohibitions during pregnancy, birth and postpartum, and menstruation. Iced drinks may be avoided; may request warm water or weak tea.

* **Food prohibitions.** (See Food beliefs and rituals.) Dairy products such as milk and cheese rarely eaten by adults, but ice cream enjoyed.

* **Food prescriptions.** (See Food beliefs and rituals.)

Symptom Management

* **Pain.** Hmong people traditionally grew and used opium for its analgesic properties. Expect same relief from Western

medicines. Medications readily accepted but instructions regarding dosage may not be followed; may continue to take more in an effort to find relief from pain. Opium still used by some Hmong in U.S.

* **Dyspnea.** Lung disease common among older Hmong, and considerable lung disease noted in opium smokers. This is accepted as part of life, and rarely complained about.

* **Nausea/vomiting.** Gastrointestinal disturbance common, and individual will freely discuss distress and request relief from symptoms.

* **Constipation/diarrhea.** Constipation occurs frequently due to poor intake of roughage but may not be reported to health care professional unless specifically asked. Diarrhea a distressful symptom and Hmong will ask for medication to control it.

* **Fatigue.** Fatigue often presenting symptom of depression.

* **Depression.** Posttraumatic stress disorder is common. Marital discord often expressed as depression in Hmong women who feel helpless to change their situation. Hmong men become depressed due to physical limitations from war injuries and sense of powerlessness since immigrating to U.S. Unemployment high for older adults due to lack of fluency in English.

* **Self-care for symptom management.** Home remedies, including cupping, coining, massage, pinching, herbs, and shaman rituals often will be tried before going to Western health care practitioners. (See Home and folk remedy section for more information.)

Birth Rituals/Care of the New Mother/Baby

* **Pregnancy care.** Prenatal care becoming more widely accepted although some mothers may not enter the system until third trimester because they are embarrassed by examinations. Hmong women have as many as 10 to 12 pregnancies. Labor can progress very rapidly for multiparous women.

* **Labor practices.** Labor practices will vary. Some women will prefer to walk about and others will lie in bed.

* **Role of the laboring woman during birth process.** Hmong women often quiet during labor although behavior

may vary. Women do not want to be examined and having multiple caretakers will increase mother's anxiety.

* **Role of the father and other family members during birth process.** Traditionally, father delivered baby by reaching under skirt of squatting mother. Full exposure of genital area not done. If problems, in-laws might assist since married couple usually lived with them. Since immigration and practice of birthing in hospitals, father usually present but assistance in labor and delivery will vary. Some men will not want to be present. Father usually at hospital and expects to make all decisions related to surgical options.

* **Vaginal vs. cesarean section.** Vaginal delivery preferred, and cesarean section often refused. Most Hmong women very small and, because of improved nutrition, babies becoming quite large. Cephalopelvic disproportion increasing, with growing need for cesarean section.

* **Breastfeeding.** Breastfeeding decreasing and bottle feeding becoming standard within Hmong community even though breastfeeding encouraged by health care professionals. Many Hmong women think American women do not breastfeed since they never see this behavior in public.

* **Birth recuperation.** New mothers remain on restricted chicken/white rice diet for 30 days after delivery. No other foods allowed during this time. Can drink warm water (no ice water) and tea made with loose tea (no tea bags). Chicken initially boiled and later may be roasted or fried, depending on mother's preferences and beliefs. Chicken must be fresh, preferably killed by father. Store-bought chicken may be used if fresh not available. Rice must be soft and white. At end of 30 days, regular diet resumed.

* **Problems with baby.** Mother-in-law assists new mother in child care and if problems occur that cannot be solved by mother or mother-in-law, male family elders will be consulted.

* **Male and female circumcision.** Neither practiced in Hmong community.

Death Rituals

* **Preparation.** Elders of family/clan will meet regarding any decisions that must be made about dying person. In Hmong culture, immediate family members and female relatives may not have exclusive decision-making power, even though they may be "next of kin" by medicolegal standards.

    Traditional Hmong religious beliefs say that when someone dies, this person will go to next world with same appearance they have at time of death. If someone dying at home, family would dress dying person in finest traditional Hmong clothing so he/she would enter next world well dressed. Considered shameful to enter next world poorly dressed or unclothed. Nurses can aid traditional families considerably by advising family when person is near death and allowing them to dress loved one in traditional clothing.

* **Home vs. hospital.** Dying either at home or hospital may be acceptable for Hmong families. Decisions always based on what they regard as best for dying person.

* **Special needs.** Do not remove amulets from body. Shaman rituals may be performed in attempt to cure dying person. These rituals must be performed in home and would be considered less effective in hospital. After death, specific rituals performed in funeral home to help send person's spirit to heaven.

* **Care of the body.** Body usually prepared for burial by family at funeral home. Family believes person will suffer if hard objects buried with body; may ask that indwelling metal plates, bullets, and shrapnel be removed from body. Person cannot be buried with buttons, zippers, or metal closures on clothing, and screws and nails will be removed from inside coffin. Traditional Hmong or Western clothing will be placed on body with extra finery placed in coffin. No Hmong metal amulets or jewelry buried with body.

* **Attitudes toward organ donation.** Traditional Hmong usually will not donate organs because they believe one of body's three spirits stays with body; therefore, body needs to stay whole. Hmong who are Christians, however, believe that

body and soul are separate and may
consent to donation.
* **Attitudes toward autopsy.**
(See Organ donation.)

Family Relationships

* **Composition/structure.** Hmong families large,
patrilineal, with well-organized hierarchy of decision making. Eldest male
relative considered head of family.
Father, followed by eldest son, head of
individual family. There are 18 Hmong
clans, and all members of clan have
same last name. All clan members
considered related and prohibited from
marrying one another, even though
close biological relationships do not
exist. Cousins in father's clan considered brothers and sisters. Sons expected to marry and bring wives to live in
family home. Daughters marry and
become part of husband's clan
although may retain birth clan's
name as surname. Men may have
more than one wife. Married Hmong
style not registered by the State. Gays
and lesbians are not acknowledged
by Hmong.

* **Decision making.** Women may express opinions, but men make final decisions. If
woman's husband is gone, eldest adult
son expected to make decisions for
mother unless she has remarried. Many
decisions made through family meetings and if head of family lives in
another state, decision making can
be an arduous process.

* **Spokesperson.** Spokesperson most likely someone who speaks English, but might not
have decision-making power.

* **Gender issues.** Women considered subservient
to men. Sons expected to always
remain with family clan and daughters
expected to leave home and join husband's clan. Most Hmong prefer sons
so their sons can care for them in their
old age. Hmong men may take second
wife if first wife does not bear sons.
Couples who have only daughters may
continue to have children in attempt
to have son.

* **Caring role.** Women are caretakers during
health and illness. When woman
considered potential mate for son, her
reputation as "hard worker" consider
part of her value as bride. After

marriage, she is expected to cook and clean for family. This role expectation persists, even though daughter-in-law may have job or go to school. Mothers-in-law take over many child-rearing responsibilities. Daughters-in-law expected to care for in-laws during illness.

* **Expectations of and for children.** Children expected to obey parents and older siblings. Decisions may be made for children regarding schooling and choice of careers. These decisions felt to be in best interest of family; individual's desires subservient to needs of family.

* **Expectations of and for elders.** Elders take on child-rearing roles when they are no longer able to work outside the home. Older people held in great respect in Hmong community and looked to for advice.

* **Expectations of adults in caring for children and elders.** See above.

* **Expectation of visitors.** When Hmong person is ill, all family members expected to go to hospital to visit. If someone doesn't go, it is thought they do not love ill person and they would be socially censured within community. Since Hmong families can be quite large and extended family members have close ties, hospital can be overwhelmed by visitors.

Spiritual/Religious Orientation

* **Primary religious/spiritual affiliation.** A recent study found that 75% of Hmong people practiced traditional religion which is animistic. Traditionalists believe that body has three souls. When someone dies, one soul goes to heaven, one stays with body, and one is reincarnated. Traditionalists practice ancestor worship and believe that ancestral spirits can protect them or can cause harm if spirits are not honored sufficiently.

    Many Hmong also practice Buddhism or Christianity with membership in various churches such as Catholic, Missionary Alliance, Baptist, Mormon, and others. Hmong who are Christians may use all traditional medical practices except shamanism which is practiced by those who retain animist beliefs.

* **Usual religious/spiritual practices.** For Hmong who retain traditional beliefs, a shaman is necessary to communicate with spirit world. During this ritual, family members gather at home and shaman rides imaginary horse to spirit world to learn why person is ill and what sacrifice required to make person well again. Healing ceremony then conducted, usually involving sacrifice of chicken, pig, or cow. Purpose of sacrificing animal is to send its spirit to other world in place of ill person's spirit that has been stolen or wandered away. Animal's spirit may also be expected to protect person from further harm. Amulets are applied at time of ceremony, intended to continue protective powers for as long as person wears them.
* **Use of spiritual healing/healers.** See above.

Illness Beliefs

* **Causes of physical illness.** Hmong believe illness can have natural or supernatural etiologies, although infectious disease etiologies are beginning to be understood. Traditional causes of illness might be soul loss or illness caused by an ancestral spirit in attempt to get person's attention and remind them that honoring ceremonies have not been sufficiently performed. Christian Hmong may have illness beliefs similar to other Westerners or feel that illness is "God's will." Hmong recently converted to Christianity may consider illness retribution from ancestral spirits for abandoning traditional ways.
* **Causes of mental illness.** There is no word for mental illness in Hmong except a word that would mean "crazy" in English. Depression common and not hidden. Some individuals who have nightmares attribute them to spirit visits from dead relatives.
* **Causes of genetic defects.** Genetic defects thought to be caused by spirits because parents did something wrong. Child accepted without stigma although marriage may be more difficult since appearance an important factor in mate selection.
* **Sick role.** Ill people expect family members to care for them. Family relationships can be strained by prolonged illnesses or

insufficient help. Patients may resist self-care practices. For example, family members may be expected to administer insulin injections.

* **Home and folk remedies.** Several methods used, intended to release evil spirits or illness-causing toxins from body. These are all similar in their primary purpose: to cause an ecchymotic area through which illness passes. Darkness of ecchymotic area also considered an indicator of seriousness of illness. These methods performed on skin over area of pain to locate pain for health care professional. Methods include:

  Cupping—cotton or tissue burned in a small glass jar. After flame is out, jar is placed over painful area and remains until air within jar has cooled, producing a vacuum and a round ecchymotic area.

  Coining—Using spoon or coin (anything with round edge), skin is stroked lightly until an ecchymotic area appears, an oval bruise with an irregular border.

  Pinching—Skin is pinched until a bruise appears, usually narrow and may be found between eyes of person with headache.

  It is common practice to puncture ecchymotic area to express blood, thereby removing toxin causing illness. Puncture often done with sewing needle, rarely sterilized. One needle may be used on several individuals.

  Herbs commonly used in Laos and still used today in U.S. Many traditional herbs not available here but some imported from Laos. Chinese herbs also popular.

* **Acceptance of procedures.** Generally, invasive procedures not well accepted. Some individuals do not want blood drawn when feeling ill because they think it will make them "too sick." Many complain if they have "too many" blood tests because they do not believe blood is regenerated. Others will request blood tests because they think they feel better afterward.

* **Care seeking.** Home remedies and traditional medicine practices often will be tried before going to Western physician, sometimes allowing disease processes to become well advanced. Preventive

medicine practices such as PAP smears gaining greater acceptance.

Health Practices

* **Concept of health.** Health equated with being able to perform expected routines. Great distress occurs when someone cannot perform usual duties.

* **Health promotion and prevention.** Not a priority in Hmong community if health promotion considered from Western perspective. Hmong practice some behaviors and avoid others because of widespread beliefs that certain Western foods or medical procedures will cause harm.

    Most Hmong parents will have children immunized. To insure compliance with immunization schedule, may need reminders by telephone or mail.

* **Screening.** Screening generally done on sick visits. Most will not come in just for screening.

Selected References

LaDu, E.B. (1985). Childbirth care for Hmong families. *Maternal Child Nursing*, 10, 382-38.

Moore-Howard, P. (1987). *The Hmong yesterday and today*. Sacramento, CA.

Westermeyer, J. (1982). DMS-III psychiatric disorders among Hmong refugees in the United States: A point prevalence study. *American Journal of Psychiatry*, 145 (2), 197-202.

Author

Sharon Johnson, RN, FNP, PhD is a graduate of University of California, San Francisco School of Nursing. Her dissertation research was "Diabetes in the Hmong Population" where she examined the emergence of diabetes in Hmong individuals including health beliefs, practices, and perspectives which influence diabetes management. She is Associate Professor at San Francisco State University and Coordinator of the Case Management in Primary Care/Family Nurse Practitioner Program.

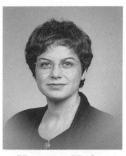

Homeyra Hafizi

Cultural/Ethnic Identity
* **Preferred terms.** Persian or Iranian
* **History of immigration/migration.**

  1950–1970 Mostly students from social elite and professional backgrounds.

  1970–1978 More diverse social background, urban and affluent, immigrated for better educational and economic opportunities.

  1979–present Left Iran because of the Islamic revolution for personal and economic security. More heterogeneous in socioeconomic and educational background. Many political exiles and forced migrants.

* **Map page.** *See Appendix C, p. 1.*

Communication
* **Major language and dialects.** Farsi (Persian) is national language. However, nearly half the country's population speaks different language or dialect, reflecting vast ethnic variation within Iran. Examples are: Turkish, Armenian Baluchi, and Kurdish. French is cultural language and English used in business.
* **Literacy assessment.** Older immigrants either do not speak English or speak in simple words and sentences. Children serve as interpreters. Difficult, especially when interpreter is young child. Use of simple terminology important.
* **Nonverbal communication.** Communication patterns, verbal and nonverbal, are influenced by hierarchy of relationships (educational and socioeconomic status). Very cautious in disclosure of personal thoughts to non-intimates. Very aware of external judgment and concerned with respectability and good appearance. To avoid embarrassment, may agree with what is said. To keep

169

social relationships smooth, outer
expressions may mask inner feelings.
Eye contact accepted between equals
and intimates. Personal space generally
closer than that of North Americans of
Northern European ethnicity. Allow
family to stay at bedside at all times.
Silence can have many meanings, from
confusion to grief, needs to be assessed
accordingly.

* **Use of interpreters.** May involve children, relatives, or friends; generally someone who can discuss more sensitive issues.

* **Greetings.** Prefer use of last name, at least on first meeting. Handshake, a slight bow, even standing when someone enters the room are appropriate greetings. Elderly must be greeted first as sign of respect. Kissing and embracing common among close relatives.

* **Tone of voice.** In presence of family, tone of voice can become loud, emotional, and animated. Among strangers, more restrained. Requests to care providers made politely.

* **Orientation toward time.** Combination of present and future. Live life to the fullest today, yet save enough to ensure safe, healthy tomorrow. Future orientation enhances effectiveness of health education and maintenance; yet fatalistic beliefs hinder complete understanding and compliance. Social time flexible, but on-time demands of dominant culture observed in business and health care arenas.

* **Consents.** Explain procedure or treatment to family spokesperson or interpreter. Some families believe in protecting loved one by disclosing only portions of reality to assure that patient does not lose hope. Yet consent should be deemed valid.

* **Privacy.** Sensitive and modest in clothing and sharing of personal information. Respect for education and authority (health care provider represents both) will allow for release of information relative to care. Concept of shame (*Haya*) is the undertone for deciding on what information is safe to share.

* **Serious or terminal illness.** Information should be presented by member of health care team who has developed trusting relationship with family. If possible, news needs to be given gradually, and never to patient while

he/she is alone. Important that eldest family member or spokesperson is present. Most Iranians believe in *tagdir* or will of God in life and death as pre-destined journey.

Activities of Daily Living

*   **Modesty.** Direct relation between modesty, age, and how traditional the individual may be. As a whole, population very modest in clothing. More comfortable with care provider of same gender. Sense of privacy as strong as modesty and ensures reserved behavior.
*   **Skin care.** Tend not to shower daily if ill since dampness and draft believed to accentuate weakness and malaise. However, important to cleanse with water after every urination or defecation.
*   **Hair care.** No particular preference.
*   **Nail care.** No particular preference.
*   **Toileting.** More inclined or even insistent to use bathroom for privacy and washing. Often prefer washing to use of toilet paper.
*   **Special clothing and amulets.** No special clothing, but try to keep body covered to avoid draft. May wear gold charm on neck chain symbolizing Islam. Occasionally, prayers are read quietly at bedside and prayer beads used.
*   **Self-care.** Family and friends an important part of care delivery to patient. Not expected that patient become too involved too early. Patient may resist self-care. Allow visitors and family to stay for extended periods of time. Find family spokesperson and look for cues to control sound level and number of visitors. Family can be an asset in patient education and recovery if approached and educated. Observe modesty and privacy with all procedures and treatments.

Food Practices

*   **Usual meal pattern.** Three meals a day. Prefer to eat in company of family. Dinner generally eaten as late as 9 or 10 pm. Rice particularly liked. Snacks mainly fruit and nuts. Tea served after each meal.
*   **Food beliefs and rituals.** Food classification of hot and cold based on humoral theory which sometimes corresponds to high and low calorie foods. Balance of the two food categories is key. For example, to treat symptoms of weakness and

vomiting after eating too many cold foods such as plums, rhubarb, cucumber, or beer, one must eat such hot foods as walnuts, onion, or honey. Women believed more susceptible to digestive problems from too much cold food. Hence, food and food combinations play very important role in balance of Iranians' social and physiological life.

* **Usual diet.** Prefer freshly bought items rather than frozen or canned. Use some dry herbs due to cost. Eating fast foods less common due to belief that they lack nutritional value. Most common starches are rice and wheat bread. Prefer soup spoon for rice rather than fork. Beans and legumes prepared in different rice mixtures and make up large part of dietary intake. Dairy products such as feta cheese, yogurt, eggs, and milk are also food staples. Meat favorites include beef, chicken, fish, and lamb. Shellfish sometimes eaten. Green leafy vegetables and fruits enjoyed and fully utilized. Fruit often served as dessert.

* **Fluids.** During illness, avoid ice cold water. Warm tea, especially sweetened with hard candy, also used. Herbal teas believed to have medicinal purposes.

* **Food prohibitions.** Strict Moslems avoid pork and alcohol. This belief has crossed cultural lines and some Armenians or Baha'is also may avoid pork. Balance of hot and cold food must be observed

* **Food prescriptions.** Again, balance of hot and cold food essential. May prefer homemade food.

Symptom Management

* **Pain.** Iranians express pain with facial grimace guarded body posture, moans, and even soft cries. Offer pain meds (may prefer IM initially), provide alternative means of relief such as warm compres Words such as throbbing, sharp/shoot ing, and biting used to describe pain. Persian phrases used to describe pain are poetic and provide vivid image of body and person's reaction to experience. In Iranian culture, body used as metaphor to express one's feel ings and thoughts, especially those no socioculturally sanctioned for public disclosure. Therefore, somatization is expression of social and personal

problems in form of bodily reactions and complaints. No difficulty understanding any of pain scales even though pain defined more in qualitative terms than quantitative. Some may believe that pain is suffering that will eventually cleanse their soul and redeem all past sins.

* **Dyspnea**. Will be very anxious during this time. Will accept medication of any nature and oxygen to control the state and to relieve accompanying fear. Give hope to patient and family that symptom of dyspnea can be controlled to a degree.

* **Nausea/vomiting.** Will readily accept medication for relief of symptoms. As complement to Western medicine, some may use herbal tea. No particular practice in reporting or cleansing after vomiting. Note: Embarrassment and shame with any bodily function that is unpleasant or considered not clean makes observance of privacy essential.

* **Constipation/diarrhea.** Any alteration in bowel function may be attributed to pathology and/or imbalance of food categories. Iranians first attempt to treat either condition with humoral remedies rather than Western medications. Medications will be accepted if other remedies not successful. Modesty does not interfere with reporting of condition to care provider.

* **Fatigue.** Consider non-physiological origins of fatigue since somatization an accepted illness behavior among Iranians. A numerical scale in this population may seem irrelevant when symptoms also serve as metaphors of sociocultural problems. Medications accepted to relieve fatigue; however, care provider cautioned to assess source of fatigue if disease pathology does not correspond.

* **Depression.** Mental illness somewhat stigmatized. Tend to pay more attention to somatic symptoms when under emotional stress. Psychopharmacology considered more effective than psychotherapy; however, more acculturated immigrants becoming more comfortable with psychotherapy. Term *Narahati* used in general to express wide range of unpleasant emotions or physical feelings such as depression, disappointment, anxiety, general feeling of fatigue, and unease. *Narahati*

expressed nonverbally in varying forms (quiet, isolated, decreased interaction), all of which are acceptable illness behaviors.

* **Self-care for symptom management.** Attempts made with home and herbal remedies to cure ailment prior to seeking medical attention. Ultimately, combination of both methods practiced to reach desired outcome. Family and friends expected to serve as care providers.

Birth Rituals/Care of the New Mother/Baby

* **Pregnancy care.** Prenatal care depends on financial stability; family provides help and support. Expectant mother encouraged to balance diet and rest adequately, and refrain from heavy work throughout pregnancy.
* **Labor practices.** Midwife or MD acceptable at childbirth. Walking prior to delivery encouraged. Generally agreeable to Lamaze classes. Fathers involved and interested in birthing experience. Offer pain relief. Showering common soon after birth.
* **Role of the laboring woman during birth process.** Depends on personality of woman. Some will moan and grunt during labor; others may get hysterical. Modesty remains controlling factor.
* **Role of the father and other family members during birth process.** More acculturated fathers take active role. Female family members are supportive and present.
* **Vaginal vs. cesarean section.** No one method preferred. Health of mother and baby defining factors.
* **Breastfeeding.** Preferred over bottle feeding. Mixed with solid food at about 4-6 months of age. Avoid prepackaged baby food. Generally do not mix breastfeeding and bottle unless mother working outside home. Breastfeeding may last as long as one year.
* **Birth recuperation.** Rest, proper diet, hygiene, and emotional ease essential. Mother, sister, or female family member and friends provide support and guidance in care of baby.
* **Problems with baby.** If baby is diagnosed with an ailment, best to speak with father of child. Always give hope and discuss methods of treatment.

* **Male and female circumcision.** Female circumcision never performed. Male circumcision either done at hospital or at later date. Male circumcision always performed; marks a period of festivity in some families.

Death Rituals

* **Preparation.** Notify head of family or spokesperson first. If medical care becomes futile, speak with head of family about options. In general, reaching a decision to make patient DNR (Do Not Resusitate) not difficult. Death seen as beginning, not end, in which mortal life gives way to spiritual existence, a cherished state of solidifying one's relationship with God. This fatalistic belief makes "death" and "letting go" easier. Assess family for individual practice.
* **Home vs. hospital.** With acute illness requiring great care, prefer hospitalization With chronic ailments, family will provide care at home.
* **Special needs.** Prefer to have family around at all times. Praying or crying softly at bedside not uncommon. Members will control noise level among themselves to provide patient with peace. Allow family to visit the body; some may decline.
* **Care of the body.** Family may decide to wash the body if no proper facilities available. Iranians may let go easier than Americans, but grieve more publicly and longer. Body not viewed after washing; therefore, embalming not practiced. Cremation not commonly practiced.
* **Attitudes toward organ donation.** Organ donation acceptable. As stated previously, discuss first with spokesperson or head of family
* **Attitudes toward autopsy.** Generally agreeable if reasoning fully explained.

Family Relationships

* **Composition/structure.** Family-oriented culture. Relationships complex and transcend many generations. Close and regular contact with friends and family a source of strength. Gay and lesbian lifestyle not tolerated except among very small number of acculturated immigrants.
* **Decision making.** Patriarchal society: thoughts

of eldest male member of both nuclear
family and extended family of utmost
importance. In some families, father is
sole decision maker.

* **Spokesperson.** Father, eldest son, eldest daughter, or eldest male family member.
Identify family spokesperson and use as
cultural and language interpreter.

* **Gender issues.** Patriarchal society: father pro-
tects and provides for family, deals
with outside world. Mother maintains
internal world and home environment.
Interfamily stress occurs when men
perceive loss of power upon relocation
to U.S., particularly with loss of
social stature.

* **Caring role.** Family plays great role in care and
support of patient. Patriarchal ideology
places mothers and other female family
members as direct care providers and
males as protectors and controllers of
outside world. Caution about general-
ization as men have been proven time
and again to assume role of care
provider with extreme finesse
and attention.

* **Expectations of and for children.** Defining
term is interdependence: mutual
dependence, respect, and responsibility. If a child is the family spokesperson
(e.g., interpreter), the family will
still expect respectful behavior from
that child.

* **Expectations of and for elders.** Age a sign of
experience and knowledge. Regardless
of kinship, all elderly respected and
cared for when self-care becomes
a concern.

* **Expectation of adults in caring for children
and elders.** Boarding schools and
nursing homes rarely utilized. Severely
mentally and physically challenged
individuals institutionalized. Sick
cared for at home if intensity and level
of care not acute.

* **Expectations of visitors.** Visitors welcomed
and helpful in recovery. If possible,
provide patient with private room to
allow for better crowd control.
Agreeable to visiting limitations if
medically necessary. Do not
underestimate power of family and
spiritual healing.

Spiritual/Religious Orientation

* **Primary religious/spiritual affiliation.**
Primarily Shiite Moslems. Other

religions include: Judaism, Christianity, Baha'i, and Zorastrian. God's will (*Tagdir*) over one's fate in life and death fosters sense of passivity and dependence on superior force. This belief weaker among more educated Iranians.

*   **Usual religious/spiritual practices.** Except for silent prayers at bedside, no other religious practices observed in hospital. Any religious practice intended for patient's return to health carried out outside hospital. May involve gathering of women for prayer at homes or helping the less fortunate, such as giving alms to needy family, both abroad and in U.S. Confessions not customary.

*   **Use of spiritual healing/healers.** Spiritual healing a function of prayers as well as family and friends' support. No spiritual healers used. No religious leaders expected to visit.

Illness Beliefs

*   **Causes of physical illness.** Health a diffuse, deeply rooted cultural concept. Health and its maintenance are continuous daily concerns dealt with mainly on subconscious level. For example, balanced intake of hot and cold food a daily consideration although not articulated day after day. Illness, however, is discussed and challenged; remedies and advice solicited. Body viewed in relation to environment: society, God, nutrition, family, etc. With presence of discomforting symptom, first inquiry is whether person ate something that did not agree with his *mezaj* (the individual's humoral temperament). If answer is no, other causes investigated. Iranians accept both Western biomedical diagnosis and their own cultural illness categories.

*   **Causes of mental illness.** Body may be metaphor for expression of fear, sadness, or issues of this nature. Assess individual patient for somatization.

*   **Causes of genetic defects.** Both scientifically and as God's punishment, depending on family's belief. Some will care for child at home and others will institutionalize, depending on child's ability to function.

*   **Sick role.** Patients assume passive role. Bad news generally kept from them.

Patient well treated by everyone and looked after. Hope never taken away.

* **Home and folk remedies.** Iranians always look for herbal and humoral cure before visiting physician; solicit advice and treatment regimens from others. Western medicine always complements home remedies and traditional cures.

* **Acceptance of procedures.** Iranians respect educated and authority figures. Health care providers well respected and listened to. Explain procedures. Problems with organ transplantation or blood transfusion rare.

* **Care seeking.** Home remedies and humoral/herbal medicine sought initially. Western medicine used in conjunction with alternative methods.

Health Practices

* **Concept of health.** Refer to Illness beliefs.
* **Health promotion and prevention.** Mainly careful of food choices, combination, preparation and compatibility of food items with each other and with individual's temperament. Herbal remedies used for symptom management and prevention. For example, mint tea used for relaxation and relief of intestinal gas and discomfort. To introduce preventive education to Iranians and solicit their cooperation, remind them that prevention always a focal point of humoral medicine.

* **Screening.** Most will agree to screening and will disclose all pertinent information.

Selected References

Hafizi, H. (1990). *Health and wellness: An Iranian outlook.* Unpublished Master's Thesis, University of California, San Francisco.

Lipson, J. G. (1992). The health and adjustment of Iranian immigrants. *Western Journal of Nursing Research,* 14(1), 10-24; discussion 24-29.

Lipson, J., & Hafizi, H. (In press) Iranians. In L. Purnell (Ed.), *Transcultural health care: A culturally competent approach.* F.A. Davis.

Pliskin, K. (1987). *Silent boundaries: Cultural constraints on sickness and diagnosis of Iranians in Israel.* New Haven CT: Yale University Press.

Author

Homeyra Hafizi, RN, MS immigrated to the U.S. from Iran at the age of 16. She is a graduate of the University of California, San Francisco School of Nursing (1991) and currently serves as the Director, Medical/Surgical Services and Behavioral Health Services at Wuesthoff Memorial Hospital in Rockledge, Florida.

CHAPTER 18

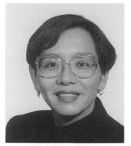
Gayle Shiba

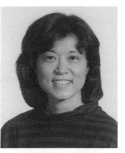
Roberta Oka

Culture/Ethnic Identity

* **Preferred term.** Japanese American.
* **History of immigration.**

1885	Early immigration from Japan to the U.S. (primarily the West Coast) and Hawaii.
1900–1910	Peak of immigration.
1924	National Origins Act barred Japanese Americans, other Asians from entering U.S. after 1924.
1942	Executive Order 9066. All persons of Japanese ancestry living in California, Washington, and Oregon forcibly moved to "relocation camps."
1950s	Renewed immigration.

The history of immigration created unique layering of generations, an integral aspect of the culture. Japanese Americans are only ethnic group to identify themselves by generation in which they were born and are distinguishable by their age, experience, language, and values. The *Issei* are first generation of Japanese Americans in U.S. *Issei* have strong sense of national identity which declines with each succeeding generation, but should not be equated with lack of strong identity with Japanese American community. The *Nisei* are second generation Japanese Americans born and educated in U.S. While appearing acculturated, *Nisei*'s feelings and attitudes rooted in Japanese culture. Third generation (*Sansei*) and fourth generation (*Yonsei*) Japanese Americans more typical of American born counterparts, less connected to Japanese culture. Japanese Americans have demonstrated ability to acculturate on many levels while maintaining viable ethnic community and identity. Recent immigrants from Japan tend to be well educated and settle in large metropolitan areas with significant Japanese/Japanese American community.

* **Map page.** *See Appendix C, p. 1.*

Communication

In general, Japanese Americans (especially older generation) may not ask many questions about their treatment or care, deferring to physician or health care professional (authorities) providing their care. Illnesses, especially those such as cancer, not freely discussed outside family. Communication influenced by cultural concepts of *enryo*, *gaman*, and *haji*. *Enryo* is self-restraint in interacting with others. May also be described as polite refusal, or polite hesitation, where patient may refuse medication or assistance if embarrassing or "inconvenient" for patient or health care professional. *Gaman* is concept related to self-control and ability to endure. Patients labeled stoic may reflect this trait. Questions should be phrased to require more than "yes" or "no" answer, as patients may not question or ask for further explanation to avoid embarrassment. Self-disclosure made only if trust has been established, and usually only when elicited. *Haji* is concept of shame, to be avoided at almost any cost, as shame reflects upon family and family name, as well as on individual.

* **Major language(s) and dialects.** Japanese, particularly with *Issei*. *Nisei* usually bilingual, with later generations speaking English only. Newly immigrated Japanese usually able to understand and speak English.

* **Literacy Assessment.** *Issei* read and understand very little English. Most *Nisei* bilingual. Later generations, *Sansei* and Yonsei, predominately literate in English.

* **Nonverbal communication.** Typically quiet and polite, will tend not to disagree or ask questions. Appear reserved and formal in new situations. Emotional outbursts discouraged. Facial expressions controlled. Respectful to elders and authority figures (nurses and physicians). Relatively little direct eye contact, especially to "superiors." Touching uncommon. Elderly may typically nod in positive manner during conversation; however, not necessarily indicative of understanding or agreement.

* **Use of interpreters.** Especially important for *Issei*. Family members preferred for translation. For privacy, discuss sensitive issues such as sex, diagnosis, etc., with close family member or same gender interpreter.

* **Greetings.** Formal in greeting (i.e., use of surname). Handshakes more common in younger generations; smile or

small bow may be used for acknowledgement.

* **Tone of voice.** Polite to speak in soft voice; direct expressions of disagreement or conflict avoided. "Face" or "saving face" an important concept and expressions of anger or loss of temper not condoned as reflects negatively upon family.

* **Orientation toward time.** Promptness important. Often early for appointments.

* **Consents.** Explain procedures clearly. Stop to elicit feedback and understanding of what is being communicated. Emphasize important details; patients may be uncomfortable asking questions for clarification. Older generation Japanese Americans more likely to agree/consent to procedure because of recommendation from health care professional.

* **Privacy.** Because of strong respect for authority, sensitive information disclosed if deemed important to care, but otherwise patient may be reluctant. Sensitive to concepts of shame and saving face.

* **Serious or terminal illness.** For older patients who speak little or no English, family may "filter" information to patient. Families may be reluctant to divulge terminal diagnosis and prognosis to patient. Consult with family members, spouse, and eldest son or daughter.

Activities of Daily Living

* **Modesty.** Very modest, particularly women. Modest even with family members, especially older people, and those of opposite sex. Gender matching ideal.

* **Skin Care.** Cleanliness and hygiene very important. Linked to belief and importance of purification of body to help restore health. Prefer daily tub baths, best in evening before bedtime.

* **Hair care.** Prefer to wash hair daily or several times per week.

* **Nail care.** Short and clean.

* **Toileting.** Use of bathroom primarily for privacy. Need to wash after toileting.

* **Special clothing/amulets.** *Issei* may use prayer beads, particularly if Buddhist.

* **Self-care.** Personal hygiene performed by patient if able. Family member, particularly spouse or elder daughter, may be

able to provide assistance, and may be preferred by patient instead of health care provider. Older adults may be more dependent on family members when ill.

Food Practices

* **Usual meal pattern.** Meals three times a day. Snacks between meals, which may consist of ethnic snacks such as rice cakes. Rice with most meals, particularly dinner. Younger generation has adopted more Western diet and meals will reflect this (less rice, for example). Food should be visually appealing.
* **Special utensils.** Chopsticks.
* **Food beliefs and rituals.** During New Year's holiday and other times of year, eating of certain food dishes (i.e., *ozoni*–soup containing *mochi*–pounded rice) thought to bring good luck/fortune and good health for family during year.
* **Usual diet.** Usually low in fat, animal protein, cholesterol, and sugar but high in salt content. Traditional protein sources— fish and soybeans with vegetables. Rice at dinner.
* **Fluids.** Primarily tea, without cream or sugar, although many drink coffee.
* **Food prohibitions.** Many are lactose/alcohol intolerant. Combinations of food such as eel and pickled plums, watermelon and crab, and cherries and milk often thought to cause illness when eaten together. These beliefs held more by older Japanese Americans.
* **Food prescriptions.** Rice gruel or porridge with pickled vegetables when ill. Hot tea when ill or for stomach ailments. Pickled plums and hot tea used to prevent constipation or maintain normal bowel function.

Symptom Management.

Generally, symptom complaints not offered by the patient. Additionally, patient may not freely ask for medications to alleviate symptoms. May delay seeking assistance for symptoms until severe.

* **Pain.** *Itami* (e-ta-mee) - to have pain. *Itai* (e-ta-ee) - it hurts. Can be stoic in expression of pain or discomfort. Offer pain medications, as ordered. Some have high pain threshold, but others may refrain from asking for medications. Older generation especially concerned about becoming addicted to medication and may refuse. Others

take medication as prescribed, preferring oral medications to injections. May refuse rectal medications.

* **Dyspnea.** Can't breathe. Will accept oxygen.
* **Nausea/vomiting.** Loss of control of bodily functions embarrassing. Some individuals or family members will clean up after an event.
* **Constipation/diarrhea.** Uncomfortable when routine disrupted. May disclose if asked. May prefer trying own remedies before taking medication. Enema last option.
* **Fatigue.** Generally will tolerate fatigue. If needed, may resort to foods thought to relieve fatigue.
* **Depression.** Psychological state or mood may not be expressed by patient due to fear of social stigma and shame.
* **Self-care for symptom management.** Older generation (*Issei*) may not respond to illness until advanced. Younger generations acknowledge illness more readily and are open to self-care for symptom management. Japanese Americans more likely to listen to health care professional than family member in pursuing self-care.

Birth Rituals/Care of the New Mother/Baby

Most Japanese Americans currently follow Westernized practices. Fathers (*Sansei*) usually present at delivery. Extended family member (usually mother's mother) assists new mother after birth of baby. Mother primary person responsible for care of child.

* **Pregnancy Care.** Prenatal care an expectation from early in pregnancy. Woman encouraged to get plenty of rest and not "overdo" during pregnancy. Mothers-to-be very health conscious, eating properly, avoiding foods and beverages that may harm baby. Generally follow prenatal care recommendations.
* **Labor Practices.** More consistent with American counterparts, unless recent immigrant. Fathers present in labor and delivery. Mother of pregnant woman may also be present. Assess for pain and offer adequate pain relief; some may not request pain medication or may refuse until pain severe.
* **Role of laboring woman during birth process.** Woman may be more assertive during labor, expressing her wishes and needs. Most women attempt to control vocal expressions

of pain or discomfort such as
screaming. Modesty important.

* **Role of the father and other family members during the birth process.** Father assumes active role during birth process if Lamaze or childbirth classes attended. If father not present during labor and delivery, presence of sister or mother of woman preferred.
* **Vaginal vs. cesarean section.** Vaginal delivery preferred.
* **Breastfeeding.** Breastfeeding, at least for some period of time, an expectation of Japanese mothers. Mothers who breast-feed may also bottle feed (i.e., one or two bottles a day). While breastfeed-ing, mother tends to be very conscious of health and diet as it benefits baby. If Japanese woman returns to work, breastfeeding often discontinued and bottle feeding implemented at that time.
* **Birth recuperation.** New mother expected to rest and recuperate for several weeks after birth. If mother's mother avail-able, she may stay with family to assist in household activities and child care. Other family members and close friends may assist in providing support (i.e., providing meals). Personal hygiene important. Mothers will bathe, shower, and perform peri-care frequently.
* **Problems with the baby.** If problem with the baby, best to consult with father before informing mother, and make certain that father or other family members are present when discussion with mother occurs.
* **Male and female circumcision.** Male circum-cision common practice, performed prior to discharge from hospital. Female circumcision not performed.

Death Rituals

* **Preparation.** Significant other (spouse) or eldest son or daughter. May encounter situations where both family and patient know that patient is seriously ill or dying, but family and patient avoid discussing situation. DNR is dif-ficult choice, decided by entire family.
* **Home vs. hospital.** For acute illnesses, hospital preferred. If choice between home and intermediate care facility, will prefer home if resources are available and can be provided at

home. With terminal diagnosis, will prefer to die at home.

* **Special needs.** Family member(s) may request to stay with patient if illness serious or terminal.

* **Care of the body.** Cleanliness important in preparing the body, and maintenance of dignity and preservation of modesty for viewing the body. Many Japanese Americans of Buddhist or Shinto faith will have the body cremated.

* **Attitudes toward organ donation.** *Issei* less likely to agree to organ donation. Strong feeling that when person dies, body should be kept intact. Do not believe in "cutting up" the body. Believe that body needs to be as it was at person's birth. *Nisei* more likely to agree; however, would respect wishes of elders if requested to give permission for organ donation from parent. *Sansei* and *Yonsei* more Westernized and would consider organ donation.

* **Attitudes toward autopsy.** *Issei* not likely to agree to autopsy; believe it not appropriate or "right." May view such an act as violation of body (see Organ donation). Younger generations more open to considering autopsy.

Family Relationships

* **Composition/structure.** Family-oriented cultural group: self subordinate to family unit. In older Japanese American families, members have well-defined roles. Family structure hierarchical, with father being head of household and major authority for family. Strong solidarity, mutual help-fulness, interdependency (*amae*), and patriarchal structure characterize family. Values include importance of family as unit, one's duty, responsibility, obligation, and maintenance of harmony. Respect for age and authority, preference for male children (though less true with later generations), and filial piety (duty and obedience to one's parents, and duty of parents to children) also strong family influences. Emphasis on family and home as opposed to individual. Gay and lesbian relationships are generally not openly acknowledged or accepted by older generations. These relationships may be seen as a shame or disgrace to the

family. Close family members may
be supportive.

* **Decision making.** Women usually involved in
decision-making process, especially in
later generation Japanese American
families; however, males tend to be
family spokespersons, usually eldest
male member present.

* **Spokesperson.** Father, eldest son, or daughter.
In younger generation families, mother
often acts as spokesperson before son
or daughter.

* **Gender issues.** Women considered subordinate
in more traditional families.

* **Caring role.** Women are primary caregivers for
family: mother, wife, daughter, or
daughter-in-law. Men are pampered;
even if sick, women tend to continue
caretaking and household activities.

* **Expectations of and for children.** Children
revered, taught to be polite, quiet, shy,
humble, and deferent to elders.
Emphasis on conforming to expectations. Emotional outbursts discouraged.
Positive reinforcement unusual as is
discussing one's own achievements.
Grown children expected to care for
parents if necessary.

* **Expectations of and for elders.** Elders respected. When elders become ill, children
and family expected to care for them
at home. While healthy, elders may
help care for household, including
children and grandchildren. Elders frequently maintain separate household
from children and grandchildren.

* **Expectations of adults in caring for children
and elders.** Sick elders traditionally
cared for at home by eldest son's family. More recent generations may place
sick elder in nursing home, although
this is difficult and may cause
much guilt.

* **Expectation of visitors.** Family member,
particularly spouse, may wish to stay at
bedside during hospitalization. Entire
family and close friends considered as
family will visit sick person. Visitors
will likely bring gift to patient (i.e.
flowers, food, etc.).

Spiritual/Religious Orientation
* **Primary religious/spiritual affiliation**
Buddhist, Shinto, and Christi
find parents of different relig
ation than children, especi
older generation families (

187

who are Buddhist, and their *Nisei* children who are Christian).

* **Usual religious/spiritual practices.** Dependent upon religious beliefs.
* **Use of spiritual healing/healers.** Depends on religious beliefs. Use of prayer and offerings prevalent in Shinto and Buddhist religions. Usually done in conjunction with traditional Western medicine.

Illness Beliefs

* **Causes of physical illness.** Older generation may not respond to illness until advanced. Younger generations more Western in their beliefs about physical illness. Chronic illness such as cancer may be attributed to *karma* and may result from bad behavior in this life or in past life, or from actions of another family member.
* **Causes of mental illness.** Thought to be loss of mental self-control caused by evil spirits, punishment for previous behavior, or not living a good life. Loss of mental self-control seen as problem of person's will power, over which they are expected to have control. Patients often seen by their families as not trying hard enough to deal with situation. Frequently not thought to be "real" illness. Social stigma and shame to one's family associated with mental illness; thus may delay or avoid seeking professional help.
* **Causes of genetic defects.** May be interpreted as punishment for parents' or family's bad behavior.
* **Sick role.** Sick cared for primarily by women; expectations for performing normal duties lifted. Sick person assumes passive role. Women, however, may continue to do household duties even while sick, although other family members may help.
* **Home and folk remedies.** Some may turn to herbal medicine to cure ailments, particularly older generation. Younger generation more Westernized, relying on Western medicine and care.
* **Acceptance of procedures.** Procedures should be explained thoroughly. Western medicine generally accepted unless contradictory to cultural or religious belief.
* **Care seeking.** May use non-traditional

sources of care in addition to Western medicine.

Health Practices

* **Concept of health.** Good health related to taking care of oneself and associated with being able to maintain independence and live disease free. Balance and harmony between oneself, society, and universe.

* **Health promotion and prevention.** Western beliefs in health promotion becoming more accepted, particularly by older generation. Younger generations more readily adopt healthy lifestyles.

* **Screening.** Health maintenance important, particularly in younger generations. *Issei* and *Nisei* may have more difficulty providing information related to screening if issues are sensitive (i.e., sex, information that may reflect negatively upon family). However, most will disclose information because of their respect for health care professionals.

Selected References

Chang, B. (1985). Asian-American patient care. In G. Henderson & M. Primeaux (Eds.), *Transcultural health care* (pp. 255-278). Menlo Park, CA: Addison-Wesley Publishing.

Hashizume, S., & Takano, J. (1983). Nursing care of Japanese American patients (Chapter 7). In M.S. Orque B. Bloch, & L. S. Monrroy (Eds.), *Ethnic nursing care: A multicultural approach* (pp. 219-243). St. Louis: C.V. Mosby.

Ishida, D., & Inouye, J. (1995). Japanese Americans. In J. Giger & R. Davidhizar (Eds.), *Transcultural nursing: Assessment and intervention* (pp. 317-345) (2nd Edition). St. Louis, MO: Mosby.

Authors

Gayle Shiba, RN, MS, PhD(c) is a doctoral candidate at the University of California, San Francisco School of Nursing studying symptom occurrence, symptom management, and self care in radiation oncology patients. She is a third generation Japanese-American whose grandparents immigrated to the United States in the early 1900s from Japan, and whose parents were relocated during World War II.

Roberta Oka, RN, DNSc is Assistant Clinical Professor at the University of California, San Francisco School of Nursing and Research Associate at the Stanford Center for Research in Disease Prevention, Stanford University School of Medicine. Her research interests are physical activity interventions in various populations. Born and raised in Hawaii, she is a third generation (*Sansei*) Japanese-American.

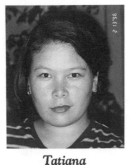

Tatiana
Reardon

Cultural/Ethnic Identity

* **Preferred term.** Korean or Korean American.
* **History of immigration.**

1903–1920   Approximately 8,000 Koreans came to U.S. and settled in Hawaii. Left Korea for many different reasons: attracted by American Christian missionaries, left country dominated by Japanese government, or famine, and seeking opportunity of plantation labor. Many were women; men brought family with them, fearing being unable to return to Korea due to Japanese control. Women also came as "picture brides." In 1905, Japan prohibited Korean emigration to Hawaii due to competition with Japanese workers already in Hawaii.

1950–1965   Approximately 17,000 Koreans entered U.S., majority being spouses of American citizens, due to War Brides Act of 1947, allowing Asian wives and children of U.S. servicemen to enter on non-quota status.

1965   Immigration Act opened gates for major wave of Asian immigration. Prior to 1965, Koreans in U.S. were few and scattered across U.S. Unlike first wave of farmers and working classes, second wave comprised those with college education and middle class backgrounds. Due to rapid industrial modernization between 1961-1971, South Korea created an economy centered on export business. To compete internationally, industry relied on low wage labor. Rice prices were low due to anti-inflation policies, initiating agricultural crisis which created influx to urban areas, causing minimal employment and population overflow. Many nurses, pharmacists, dentists, and physicians came to U.S. between 1965 and 1977.

* **Map page.** *See Appendix C, p. 1.*

Communication

* **Major language and dialects.** Korean.
* **Literacy assessment.** Elder first generation Korean Americans may or may not speak English; if they speak English, may be limited to few phrases. May understand more than they can speak. If intimidated or unsure of stranger's motives, may appear unable to speak or understand any English. Most accurate assessment of understanding is by directly asking patient or family member. Ability to speak English does not necessarily equate with capability of reading and writing English. Many older Koreans have learned English from family members and from media such as television.
* **Nonverbal communication.** When comfortable with each other (such as family members), touching, friendly pushing, hugging accepted. Among strangers, however, touching considered disrespectful unless for examination purposes; makes Korean patient uncomfortable. Considered rude to direct sole of shoe or foot toward another person. Direct eye contact infrequent from patient to nurse unless patient is comfortable with nurse. Patient may frequently look/glance at nurse when nurse not looking, part of assessment of "this nurse/stranger," and way for patient to become more comfortable. Personal space frequently shared with each other, but not appropriate for stranger to step into unless needed, as with examination. Silence usually accepted as quiet, tranquil time; may meditate or pray. Silence equated with being alone. Silence will also exist among strangers. With each other, Koreans very excitable and animated in communication; silence usually uncommon.
* **Use of interpreters.** Important to use family members as much as possible as patient is more comfortable. If no family

member present and interpreter available, realizing that stranger speaks same language will relieve patient uneasiness. Gender should not be heavily weighed as factor since interpreters are introduced in professional setting. When patient elderly, the gender of interpreter is not important as long as respect established.

* **Greeting.** Use Mr./Mrs./Ms and last name unless patient requests otherwise. Respect toward elders and authority figures is constant, demonstrated by quick quarter-bowing. Doctors well respected within Korean community; mixed feelings toward nurses (in old days in Korea, nurses only required elementary education; present day level of preparation not experienced before).

* **Tone of voice.** Tone has wide variety of pitches with emphasized loudness on what speaker finds relevant or important. Strangers may interpret normal Korean language conversation as arguing or bickering. Commands will be vocalized differently, depending on whether directed to elder or younger individual: louder and authoritative toward younger generation and quieter and friendlier toward elders.

* **Orientation toward time.** Generally, time important and punctuality normal. Past regarded as important integral part of one's identity and where life's lessons are learned. Present is all about living and carrying on with life; family relations with peaceful interactions are focus. Future perceived, but not relied on heavily for fear of jeopardizing its existence (common for elders); many enjoy thinking of present. Fate commonly accepted; in life, everything happens for a reason.

* **Consents.** Procedures should be explained in clear, understandable manner; time to think or review may be requested. Do not rush or make patient feel pressured.

* **Privacy.** Pride and shame prevalent within Korean community; if patient feels embarrassed, will be reluctant to disclose information. Be sensitive to words and facial expressions when explaining some aspect of care or diagnosis. Assess if patient wants family member present. Trust must be established for patient to reveal personal or

pertinent information. Also, what may
not be viewed as private issue by nurse
may be significantly private to patient.
* **Serious or terminal illness.** Family, preferably
spokesperson, should be informed of
diagnosis and this person or family
will then inform patient of prognosis.
Family will join as a unit and
prepare together.

Activities of Daily Living
* **Modesty.** Very modest, especially women; offer
robes and hospital pants to both male
and female patients. Frequently,
patients feel temperature is too cold,
and prefer multiple layers of clothing,
as well as foot coverings. Elders frequently wear thermal undergarments.
* **Skin care.** Very clean, probably prefer sponge
bathing when in hospital, thus need
many washcloths. Patients do not like
to feel dirty; may perform peri-care
often. Common practice is to rub skin
with rough cloth while bathing, helping with exfoliation of dead skin.
* **Hair care.** Depends on level of dryness or oili-
ness of hair. Many older women do not
shampoo daily; may only wash hair
once or twice per week.
* **Nail care.** Prefer very clean and well-trimmed
nails; frequently will trim or even out
any breaks or remove hangnails, etc.
* **Toileting.** Prefer to use bathroom for
privacy and may also wish to perform
peri-care.
* **Special clothing/amulets.** Usually minimal
jewelry; may wear religious symbols
such as Christian representations.
* **Self-care.** Younger patients perform own
hygiene, but older patients, even if
able, may have family members
perform care. Usually family members
will not ask, but just perform care;
generally accepted as duty of children.

Food Practices
* **Usual meal pattern.** May or may not eat three
meals a day, but will frequently have
snacks, usually fruit. Dinner usually
main meal and time when most family
members can gather together and
interact. Usually will eat until hunger
satisfied; thus, if breakfast was big,
lunch may or may not be eaten.
* **Special utensils.** Usually eat with chopstick
and big soup spoons.

* **Food beliefs and rituals.** Cold fluids such as iced beverages usually not welcome; Koreans relate cold with imbalance or causing illness.

* **Usual diet.** Korean diet high in fiber and spicy, consisting primarily of rice, bean curd, vegetables, fruits, seafood, lean meats, occasionally pork, pickled vegetables with ever popular *Kim-chee* being standard. Many meals consist of soups or broth prepared with plenty of vegetables, noodles, and small portion of meat; soups usually preferred spicy. Hot sauces made from peppers and soybeans also frequently present with meals.

* **Fluids.** One popular type of drink prepared by boiling large kernels of corn, straining corn, and then storing water in refrigerator. Elder Koreans do not like water straight from tap, fearing contamination; therefore, may boil water and store in refrigerator before drinking. Many fluids consumed in form of broth and soups.

* **Food prohibitions.** Dairy products not often in Korean diet; many Koreans lactose intolerant, therefore tend to avoid cheese, milk, etc. Cold fluids not popular, nor is anything outside of usual diet. See Pregnancy Care for diet of pregnant women.

* **Food prescriptions.** Ginseng commonly used to relieve cold symptoms. When individuals have colds, common to add fresh slices of ginger, lemon, and a big spoonful of honey to a cup of black tea. Various soups considered to have therapeutic effects when ill; onions, garlic, and spices thought to help one breathe better by cleansing sinuses.

Symptom Management

* **Pain.** *Ah-poom nida* means much pain, and *chegesso* or *chegetta* means "I could die" (not literally, but frequently stated for dramatic purposes or exaggeration, equating to pain). May be stoic, especially men; thus health care provider should frequently ask how bad pain is rather than using pain scale (may be too intangible). Some may be very expressive and frequently will moan or flail about; not unusual to be dramatic when in hospital, especially when family members present. Pain medications not used frequently for fear of

195

addiction or complications. When
pain medications are used, PO and IV
routes usually preferred to IM, viewed
as being invasive.

* **Dyspnea.** *Soomi cham-nida* means shortness of
breath or dyspnea. Will be very wor-
ried and try to breathe faster and deep-
er; oxygen may not be welcomed due
to fear of progressive disease or worsen-
ing of condition.

* **Nausea/vomiting.** *Toe-ha guess soom nida*
means nausea. Usually will tell RN
after vomiting due to embarrassment
or desire to vomit in private. May not
want anti-nausea medication.

* **Constipation/diarrhea.** *Byuenbi* means constipation and *sul-sa* means diarrhea. Due
to modesty, may not inform RN unless
severe; yet will be very concerned if
usual regime changes. May take
medications to assist with defecation,
preferring oral medications to enemas
or suppositories.

* **Fatigue.** *(Pee-lo haum-nida)* May not report
fatigue, but may want to avoid ADL's
and ambulation. Will probably nap frequently, but will not want to use medications to counteract fatigue.

* **Depression.** *(Chim-ool haumnida)* Due to
common view of depression or any
mental health problem as shameful,
will not reveal depression to RN unless
asked. Patient may hint through nonverbal communication and posture. If
depression reported and acknowledged,
may be hesitant to use anti-depressive
medications.

* **Self-care for symptom management.** May
not perform self-care for symptom
management, depending on level of
acceptance and how much family
provides and assists.

Birth Rituals/Care of the New Mother/Baby

* **Pregnancy care.** If affordable, prenatal care
expected. Many women place great
importance on following exactly what
health care provider recommends.

Diet an important factor during
pregnancy. Avoidance of cold soups or
liquids emphasized (cold liquids associated with potential harm to pregnancy
and also associated with *yin* and *yang*
concept). Seaweed soup popular,
known to cleanse blood and assist with
milk production. If following folk
beliefs, certain animal foods are

avoided such as chicken, crab, eggs, duck, and rabbit because they may harm infant's character or appearance. Dairy products normally not part of Korean diet; therefore, important to teach regarding use of non-dairy substitutes.

Rest promoted throughout and after pregnancy; some view activity restriction as important and will hire household help.

* **Labor practices.** Birthing attendants can be anyone in family; husband now encouraged to participate in pregnancy, whereas in earlier times he had minimal involvement. Water pitchers should be filled with lukewarm water, no ice. Showering may be avoided due to exposure to cold; thus sponge bathing common. Pain control may or may not be viewed as important; some may interpret use of pain relief medications as potential harm to baby.

* **Role of the laboring woman during birth process.** In earlier times, women expected to be strong and tolerate labor under worst circumstances. Today women encouraged to be active and less passive; vocalization during labor common although older in-laws or family members may discourage shouting or outcry as representing aggressiveness.

* **Vaginal vs. cesarean section.** Preference favors health of baby; parents choose whatever would decrease negative health implications for infant.

* **Breastfeeding.** Breastfeeding may or may not be favored; education needed to supplement what family members teach mother. If breastfeeding chosen, duration, freezing, and storage of milk, breast pumping, etc., may not be considered important; thus, teaching needed as to methods for incorporating feeding schedule in everyday activities and keeping milk fresh and safe for baby.

* **Birth recuperation.** Usually birth recuperation emphasized as important. Rest is primary focus, unless economic obligations preclude. Family members expected to assist mother with meal preparations and house cleaning so she can focus on baby.

* **Problems with baby.** Tell family spokesperson first, such as father of baby, as soon as

diagnosis or illness noted. Mother may view any problem as her fault for incorrect behavior. Important to reassure her as well as family that, whatever the situation, no one should be blamed.

* **Male and female circumcision.** Females not circumcised. When pros and cons of male circumcision presented to parents, usually choose to have circumcision due to decreased risk of infection.

Death Rituals

* **Preparation.** Imminence of death should be told to spokesperson, who will relay information to family. They will unite and prepare themselves and patient for death.

* **Home vs. hospital.** Since more services and knowledge available today, family may choose to have patient remain in hospital if seen as in the patient's best interest. Many family members may be working or attending school; therefore, lack of 24-hour care may prevent bringing patient home.

* **Special needs.** Family mourning and crying not unusual. To outsider, mourning style may be over-dramatized but this excitement not unusual and is accepted as normal. Chanting, incense burning, praying, etc., may be incorporated into hospital environment.

* **Care of the body.** Family will want to spend time with patient after death and cleansing of the body may or may not be requested. Cremation not common; associated with destroying soul or spirit.

* **Attitudes toward organ donation.** Usually organ donation considered negatively and family may refuse. Associated with tampering of body/soul/spirit.

* **Attitudes toward autopsy.** If sudden death occurs and reasons not known, family may consider; however, attitude is same as toward organ donation.

Family Relationships

* **Composition/structure.** Family considered very important. Self esteem gained through family identification, holding honor, and approval from other community groups. Life goals focused on fulfilling family roles and obligations. Cohesion, interdependence, relations in order of hierarchy, and harmony

considered important factors in successful family. Expression of love indirect. Families both nuclear and extended; not uncommon to have up to three generations living in household. Low tolerance of gay/lesbian members due to unfamiliarity; much teaching and awareness of gay/lesbian community needed within Korean culture to decrease negativity and promote awareness and acceptance.

*   **Decision making.** In past, Korean culture strongly patriarchal. Today, decision making more family-focused, although husband, father, or eldest son may have final say.

*   **Spokesperson.** Husband, father, or eldest son/daughter act as spokesperson.

*   **Gender issues.** Both men and women may be viewed as financial support for family; yet traditional roles still exist. Women may be viewed as caretaker of home and children with primary decision-making responsibilities province of husband/father.

*   **Caring role.** Usually women responsible for actual bedside care. Patient care may be so complete as to hinder basic needs such as ambulation; many think ambulation on first postoperative day aggressive and wrong.

*   **Expectations of and for children.** Children usually reared to be obedient and orderly, especially outside of home environment. Independence not promoted early; family considered very important. Education a number one goal and college education a must.

*   **Expectations of elders.** Elders treated with utmost respect. Welcomed to live with family for duration of their lives. Common to view elders living with children and grandchildren as reward for everything elders have provided during their life. Grandparents frequently care for grandchildren while parents work.

*   **Expectations of adults in caring for children and elders.** Preferred setting of care for children and elders is home; however, if unable to care for elders at home for various reasons, may place in nursing home, viewed as negative choice. Many individuals in a "sandwich generation" situation, caring for their children as well as their parents.

* **Expectation of visitors.** Visitors outside family will frequently come to see patient as sign of respect, especially if patient is elder; usually welcomed warmly. When family members taking care of hospitalized patient, will sleep in a cot next to bed. Will also bring or prepare Korean food and feed patient.

Spiritual/Religious Orientation
* **Primary religious/spiritual affiliation.** Immigrants predominately Christian. Oldest religion in Korea is shamanism or spirit worship. Souls/spirits and negativity can be readjusted by having good relationship with shamanism. Taoism, Buddhism, and Confucianism practiced in Korea before Christianity.
* **Usual religious/spiritual practices.** Chanting and praying common. Confucian and Buddhist traditions mixed with shamanism prevalent among many Koreans. Not uncommon to have mixture of faiths within one household.
* **Use of spiritual healing/healers.** May try to drive out evil spirit by hiring a moodang, who tries to discover cause of evil spirit and how to get rid of it.

Illness Beliefs
* **Causes of physical illness.** Buddhist doctrine views life as birth, old-age, illness, and death; therefore, illness and death accepted. However, many raised to view illness as result of some sort of bad luck or misfortune; many believe that it some sort of payback for something they've done wrong in past (*karma*). Therefore, may be stoic as unable to change course of luck. Helplessness, denial, and depression may result. Illness formerly believed to be caused by imbalance of hot and cold and/or disharmony in nature and environment.
* **Causes of mental illness.** See above. Also, disruption of spiritual self may be viewed as reason; shamanism may come into play.
* **Causes of genetic defects.** Parents may feel responsible, having done something wrong. Some may favor caring for child at home while others will institutionalize.
* **Sick role.** Common for family member to behave as very ill, possibly worse than they actually feel, normal for this

culture. Again, outsiders may view patient as being dramatic but this behavior is appropriate in Korean culture. Pain assessment difficult due to outward appearance of great suffering even though pain may be mild. Passivity expected and family takes care of patient's basic needs.

* **Home and folk remedies.** Herbal therapies widely used. *Hanyak* means herbal medicine, and every city with large Korean population has herbal medicine shops. Ginseng also popular; if home dosaging (usually in form of tea) does not work, may seek a *hanui* or a traditional herbal medicine doctor, who prescribes herbs and may also do acupuncture and other traditional remedies which may leave marks on skin (e.g., ecchymosis with cupping).

* **Acceptance of procedures.** Clear, slow explanation is key toward patient feeling comfortable with material presented. If patient feels that nurse is rushed or demanding, may lose trust. May also feel need to discuss even simple procedures with family members; allow time for conferring.

* **Care seeking.** May believe in both Eastern and Western medicine and seek care from both simultaneously. Some view surgery as separate entity or illness in itself.

Health Practices

* **Concept of health.** Being healthy seen as having harmony or balance between soul and physical being. Health defined as being free of symptoms and able to balance all aspects of life: raising family, providing or being provided for financially, living in warm home, etc.

* **Health promotion and prevention.** Keeping balance within all factors of one's life is main goal for maintaining and promoting health. Korean diet primarily healthy foods: rice, vegetables, fruits, lean meats, and bean curd, although high level of sodium in such staple foods as *Kim-chee*, pickled vegetables, hot sauces, and soy sauce. Exercise popular with younger generation; older generation frequently uses walking as daily activity. Health promotion within this cultural community should be focused on reducing sodium in diet.

* **Screening.** Screening not opposed if explained thoroughly. Doctors viewed as very

intelligent in this culture; thus, if
patient asked appropriately, resistance
minimal. Gynecologic screening better
received if performed by female health
care provider.

Selected References

Kee-Joung Y. P., & Peterson, L. M. (1991). Beliefs,
practices, and experiences of Korean women in relation
to childbirth. *Health Care for Women International, 12,*
261-269.

Kim, M. T. (1995). Cultural influences on depression in
Korean Americans. *Journal of Psychosocial Nursing and
Mental Health Services, 33*(2), 13-18.

Nilchaikovit, T., Hill, J. M., & Holland, J. C. (1993).
The effects of culture on illness behavior and medical
care: Asian and American differences. *General Hospital
Psychiatry, 15,* 41-50.

Pritham, U. A., & Sammons, L. N. (1993). Korean
women's attitudes toward pregnancy and prenatal care.
Health Care for Women International, 14, 145-153.

Takaki, R. (1989). *Strangers from a different stone: A
history of Asian Americans.* New York: Penguin Books.

Author
Tatiana Reardon, RN, BS is a masters student at the
University of California, San Francisco School of
Nursing in the Adult Nurse Practitioner Program. In
addition, she is working on the cardiology/cardiothoracic
medical surgical unit at the Medical Center at
University of California, San Francisco. Her mother
immigrated from Korea in 1965 after marrying her Irish
father, and Tatiana was born in the United States.

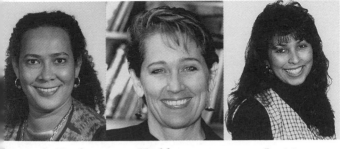

ereza de Paula   *Kathleen Laganá*   *Leticia Gonzalez-Ramirez*

Mexican Americans demonstrate wide diversity in health beliefs and practices, influenced by level of education, socioeconomic status, generation, time spent in U.S., and degree of affinity to traditional Mexican culture. Those from urban settings with higher levels of education tend to have more exposure to Western medical practices; also more likely to be bicultural, selectively maintaining certain Mexican cultural factors. Diversity within this population makes it difficult to generalize about Mexican American health beliefs and practices. Mexican American health beliefs and practices discussed here from traditional perspective, understanding that individuals may subscribe to all, some, or (possibly) none of these. Mexican Americans are defined as those individuals reporting Mexican cultural heritage, who self-identify as permanent residents of U.S., regardless of legal residency status.

Cultural/Ethnic Identity

* **Preferred term.** "Hispanic" was used in 1980 U.S. Census to collectively describe all individuals of Mexican, Cuban, Central American, Spanish, and Puerto Rican heritage. Chicano (specific to Mexican Americans) and La Raza have been replaced by Latino as an expression of Latin solidarity. Mexican American is a common self-identification. While recognizing their Mexican heritage, many prefer to be identified as American. Difficulty in finding a "preferred term" that fits all people of Mexican cultural heritage accents diversity of this ethnic group.

* **History of immigration.** War between U.S. and Mexico (1846-1848) resulted in loss of nearly half of Mexico's territory. Mexican inhabitants of ceded lands offered U.S. citizenship with promise of property rights. Some 80,000 Méxicanos living in new U.S. territory were ancestors of today's fourth, fifth, and sixth generation Mexican

Americans. Many assimilated into general Anglo population, while others continued to live in isolated cultural enclaves of Southwest.

Mexican immigration accounts for majority of today's Mexican American population. Between 1900 and 1990, 2.5 million Mexicans legally crossed into U.S. Far greater and undetermined numbers have come without documentation. Largely unsupervised border between two countries, need for cheap U.S. labor, and political and economic instability in Mexico attracted immigrants to U.S. in search of better life.

Late 1800s   Laborers imported to build railroads.

1900–1910   Heterogeneous refugees of revolution from northeastern border states of Mexico.

1911–1920   WWI labor shortages in U.S. Recruited Mexicans who were exempt from federal legislation barring Chinese labor recruitment.

1921–1930   Endemic poverty in Mexico and Christian religious persecutions. Demographic profiles like earlier European immigrants. From Texas and California, fanned out over U.S. and laid foundation for generational growth of Mexican American population.

1931–1940   Great Depression: repatriation and deportation back to Mexico (estimated at 458,000). By 1940, there were more U.S.-born Mexican Americans than Mexico-born.

1941–1964   Bracero Farm Labor Program: especially during WWII and Korean war.

1964–1986   Establishment of border *maquiladora* districts in Mexico for foreign-owned factories. More people at border created job shortages there and increased undocumented immigration, with increased numbers of single women.

1986–present. 1986 Reform and Control Act increased family reunification. More skilled persons settled in urban centers and competed for jobs in service industry. Less migrant activity.

*   **Map page.** *See Appendix C, p. 2.*

Communication

* **Major language(s) and dialects.** Some speak Spanish exclusively. Majority bilingual (Spanish/English) or monolingual (English). Many indigenous languages in Mexico. Spanish may be second language. Differences in word usage depending on individual's home region.

* **Literacy assessment.** Great diversity in educational level. Number of individuals with college education increasing annually. Monolingual Spanish speaking does not equate with lack of formal education. On average, Mexican Americans younger, poorer, and have fewer years of formal education than Anglo Americans. First generation women who do not work outside home tend to be less fluent in English. Oral English skills may exceed skill in reading and writing English. Important to assess reading skills and provide clear verbal and visual instructions and demonstrations.

* **Nonverbal communication.** Nonverbal communication strongly influenced by *respeto* (respect). Direct eye contact frequently avoided with authority figures such as health care providers or those with perceived class differences. Family members may demonstrate *respeto* by standing when provider enters room. Silence sometimes shows lack of agreement with plan of care. Touch by strangers generally unappreciated and can be very stressful or perceived as disrespectful. However, therapeutic touch an integral part of traditional healing. Handshaking considered polite and usually welcomed. *Simpatía* (social behavior promoting smooth relationships) may or may not translate to rapport.

* **Use of interpreters.** Translators fluent in English and person's preferred language should be arranged. Written information should be in person's language of choice. Use of family members or individuals not knowledgeable about health care can lead to miscommunication about complex or sensitive issues. Generally, same gender translators preferred.

* **Greetings.** Considered respectful to address individuals formally. Formal Spanish

usted should be used, especially with elders and married women. Children included in introductions. With establishment of rapport over time, providers may be permitted to be less formal. Usually very warm and expressive with family and close friends. Embracing common.

* **Tone of voice.** Respectful and polite, frequently complementary, usually reserved in formal settings.
* **Orientation toward time.** Traditionally present–oriented. Time viewed as relative to situation. This flexibility allows for feeling of punctuality even when 15–20 minutes late. Social time more present-oriented than business time. More acculturated or bicultural Mexican Americans demonstrate increased concern for punctuality in themselves.
* **Consents.** Informed consent requires clear explanation of health situation, with full array of recommended interventions, from which informed choice is made. Individuals may ask for provider's opinion. Language preference, optimum translation, and literacy levels must be considered. As noted earlier, much diversity exists in these areas among Mexican Americans.
* **Privacy.** Familialism influences privacy needs. Most sensitive issues, including health issues, kept within family. Immediate family members may serve as referents for individual concerns. Increasingly, women do not share information about contraceptive activities with family. Males disclose less often. Self-disclosure to same gender individuals usually more comfortable.
* **Serious or terminal illness.** Family may want to protect an ill family member from knowledge of seriousness of illness, based on strong belief in mind-body connection and concern that worry will worsen health status. Information about gravity of illness usually handled by family spokesperson (often older daughter or son).

Activities of Daily Living
* **Modesty.** Traditionally, Mexican Americans receive health care from women. Modesty especially pronounced in women, best respected by providing female health care providers for

sensitive physical examinations. Male physicians generally accepted, but comfort level greatly enhanced by those who demonstrate sensitivity to issue of modesty. Try to respect privacy whenever possible; allow family members to assist with ADLs. Always cover patient during physical examination and explain procedures in advance. Presence of non-essential persons in examination room discouraged.

* **Skin care.** Mexican Americans bathe daily, pay close attention to grooming and appearance. Society considered very critical of appearance. Presentation of self probably related to respect for family's reputation.

* **Hair care.** Normally, hair washed daily. Traditionally, women wear hair long, braided during times of illness or bedrest.

* **Nail care.** Clean and well kept.

* **Toileting.** Privacy essential when using bathrooms. Bedpans and bedside commodes disliked as unclean and immodest.

* **Special clothing or amulets.** Personal articles may be brought to hospital to ensure success of hospitalization and good health. Religious items, such as rosaries, frequently kept on person. Postpartum women instructed to cover their backs and to wear a *faja*, wide cloth band wrapped around abdomen. Respect for cultural elders may enhance use of special items among relatively acculturated Mexican Americans.

* **Self-care.** Traditional belief that health is controlled by environment, by fate (*distino*), and by will of God (*las manos de Dios*). Clients may rely on health care providers and family members for care. Patients will perform own hygiene when asked and if able. Traditionally, family members actively involved in ADLs. Many believe self-care can adversely affect recovery. Hospital environment or policy such as restrictive visiting hours, open disapproval of traditional caregiving activities, or patient activity expectations, such as early ambulation, that are in direct opposition to traditional beliefs and practices, can impede caregiving role of family.

Food Practices

* **Usual meal pattern.** Mexican Americans usually have three meals a day. Lunch and dinner bigger than breakfast. Prefer to eat meals together, but U.S. lifestyle interferes with this in more acculturated and nuclear families. When extended family lives in same household, meals frequently prepared by non-working grandmother, facilitating regularity in meal times. In traditional agricultural settings, men may eat first. If snacks eaten between meals, tend to be of poor nutritional quality.

* **Food beliefs and rituals.** Traditional food beliefs, traced to Galen's humoral theory, based on belief that body's four humors, blood, phlegm, yellow bile, and black bile, must be kept in balance using qualities of heat, cold, moisture, and dryness. Certain illnesses considered hot or cold states and treated with foods that complement those states. Humoral theory does not refer to temperature of foodstuff but to effects certain substances thought to have on body. Patients may refuse certain food due to these beliefs.

* **Usual diet.** Traditionally, fresh natural ingredients. Processed foods distrusted and disliked aesthetically. Although teens appear to favor fast food, many parent report that these less nutritious foods are cost prohibitive. Whenever possible, family should be encouraged to bring preferred foods from home.

    Beans and *tortillas* staples in most meals; rice also frequently included. Corn *tortillas* preferred over flour *tortillas*.

    Fresh fruits and vegetables. Prefer vegetables cooked. Tomatoes widely used for variety of sauces and included in *salsa* with onions, cilantro, chilies varying degrees of spiciness. Chilies also stuffed with highly nutritious ingredients. Nopales cactus another favorite vegetable.

    Servings of meat modest because of cost and fat content. Intake in U.S. is higher than in Mexico, possibly because of higher standard of living here. Chicken is used to make *caldo de pollo*, soup given to recuperating individuals.

* **Fluids.** Fluids used to treat some of symptoms identified by hot and cold theory.

Abundant fresh, clean drinking water considered to be health promoting. Herbal teas used for their medicinal properties.

* **Food prohibitions.** Most food prohibitions related to belief in humoral theory. Processed food discouraged. Some Catholics prefer not to eat meat on Fridays, especially during Lent.

* **Food prescriptions.** Soup (*caldo de pollo*) and herbal teas frequently administered to speed recuperation. *Yerba Buena* used as general tonic; chamomile used to treat gastric upset, especially for colic in newborn. Milder, lighter foods frequently encouraged during illness and recuperation, with less consumption of chiles or meats.

Symptom Management

* **Pain.** Patients tend not to complain of pain. Assess pain by nonverbal cues. Mexican Americans prize inner control and self-endurance. For some men, expressing pain shows weakness and possible loss of respect. Expression of pain socially more acceptable in women; however, stoicism common.

* **Dyspnea.** Tendency to feel that something is very wrong if oxygen required.

* **Nausea/vomiting.** Symptom will be disclosed if asked. See discussion of dehydration below.

* **Constipation/diarrhea.** Will be disclosed if asked. Some believe diarrhea beneficial purging of cause of illness and may not agree with use of medications to stop it. Information about dehydration required; especially important in management of children with diarrhea. Herbal teas well accepted as healing agents and may be effective means of correcting dehydration. Traditional diet usually adequate to avoid constipation.

* **Fatigue.** In Mexico, siesta is rest period that occurs after midday meal. Some in U.S. choose to rest after lunch and in areas with large percentage of Mexican Americans, this practice continues in abbreviated form. Major difference with lifestyle in Mexico is 30 to 60 minute noontime work break in U.S. that does not allow time for return home. Many women report exhaustion, related to multiple roles (domestic work, motherhood, and outside

work). Presence of grandmother in household instrumental in decreasing workload on Mexican American women.

* **Depression.** Not easily disclosed, seen as mental illness, sign of weakness, and embarrassment to family. Depression most common response to stress in Mexican Americans.

* **Self-care for symptom management.** Informal health care system in Mexico and other Latin countries includes self-medication. In theory, prescriptions required for all medications such as antibiotics and steroids, but in practice sale of drugs is uncontrolled. Pharmacist is, in effect, physician-surrogate.

Birth Rituals/Care of the New Mother/Baby

Children highly valued and protected. Motherhood role seen by many women as most important social role woman can achieve. Because of this, time surrounding pregnancy and birth especially rich in traditional beliefs and practices.

* **Pregnancy care.** Barriers to prenatal care include fear of health care system, financial constraints, and lack of transportation. Many women believe pregnancy not an illness and prenatal care unnecessary. Others seek prenatal care for reassurance of fetal well-being. Early and regular prenatal care usually associated with higher socioeconomic and educational levels and acculturation to Western health care belief system. Paradoxically, Mexican American women with late or no prenatal care experience have surprisingly healthy birth outcomes.

    Many women from lower socioeconomic levels attend clinics staffed by nurse practitioners, physicians or nurse midwives, with physicians and midwives supervising deliveries. Women with adequate financial resources generally choose obstetricians.

    Familialism (strong attachment to nuclear and extended family) provides supportive and respectful environment for pregnant women. Women who are attentive mothers are highly respected. Expectant mothers discouraged from heavy work and harmful activities such as smoking, drinking, or drug use. Encouraged to frequently rest, walk, eat well, and get plenty of sleep. Finances permitting, less acculturated women readily relinquish other roles to insure healthy birth outcome. More acculturated women with outside jobs report more role conflict. Common for grandmothers to move into nuclear family homes during last weeks of pregnancy and for weeks following delivery (sometimes coming from great distances). Grandmother or other female family members assume domestic roles and assist pregnant woman and new mother in health maintenance and restoration. Prenatal care has very broad meaning to Mexican American women, including informal home care from family members. Pregnant women protected from folk illnesses such as *Mal de ojo* (evil eye), *susto* (fright), and *antojos* (cravings). See Illness Beliefs. Often, folk medicine carried from Mexico by mothers and grandmothers and used within confines of extended family. This information usually not shared with practitioners. More acculturated women sometimes reluctantly report belief in these practices as unexplainable but effective.

* **Labor practices.** Walking recommended to ensure quick birth. One folk belief is that inactivity will result in loss of amniotic fluid, causing fetus to stick (*se pega*) to uterus. Fear of unnecessary or dangerous medical interventions, separation from family members, and loss of physical privacy leads many women to labor at home for much of labor with supportive female family members, arriving at hospital in advanced labor. More acculturated women, especially those lacking labor support from experienced women, generally come to hospital earlier and rely on health care providers for labor support.

* **Role of the laboring woman during birth process.** Historically, Mexican American woman portrayed as *la Sufrida*, a passive participant, expected to suffer in silence and deliver child to her husband. This is outmoded and stereotypical. Laboring women seen as strong and forebearing participants in natural process. Family members usually reinforce this belief, helping woman through periods of fearfulness. Many

Mexican American women supplement family support with childbirth classes, making them more informed and active participants.

* **Role of the father and other family members during birth process.** Traditionally, men not present at delivery. Usually wait in another place. Sisters, mothers, mother-in-laws, or grandmothers assist and coach during labor. More acculturated couples attend childbirth preparation classes which encourage active participation of father. Except for father of baby, men not present during active labor and delivery, but may be part of large extended group of friends and family present during early labor. Important to support woman's preferences in labor assistants. Asking about this in private demonstrates sensitivity to concept of *simpatía*.

* **Vaginal vs. cesarean section.** Normal spontaneous vaginal delivery preferred. Mexican American women fear unnecessary cesarean delivery, see surgery as life threatening.

* **Breastfeeding.** Most women breastfeed. Formula promotion in Latin America has led some women to believe breastfeeding less nutritious.

* **Birth recuperation.** Traditional 40-day period of recuperation called *la cuarentena*. Women cared for by other women, but expected to care for newborn. Domestic chores taken on by female relatives or friends. New mothers discouraged from taking showers for several days, also discouraged from getting out of bed for first few hours after birth and then only to use bathroom. Light foods provided, including *caldo de pollo*, herbal teas, and *tortillas*. Beans avoided.

    Life in U.S. rarely offers luxury of *la cuarentena*. Economic needs and separation from extended family lead many women to resume domestic or work activities within first two weeks. Some women feel *la cuarentena* unduly restrictive and old-fashioned, but make efforts to comply to some degree as show of respect to women who assist.

* **Problems with baby.** Traditionally, consultation with head of household expected as felt that new mothers should be sheltered from worry. Maternal dietary restrictions protect newborn infant

from illness or discomfort (e.g., chilies and beans). Family may need information on risks of dehydration (e.g., *Caida de Mollera* and diarrhea. See Illness Beliefs.) and helpful Western medical interventions. Infants sometimes treated with herbal teas, such as *manzanilla* (chamomile) for colic.

* **Male and female circumcision.** Circumcision in males or females not practiced in traditional Mexican American culture. However, male circumcision sometimes practiced by more acculturated families.

Death Rituals

* **Preparation.** Extended families obligated to attend to sick and dying and pay their respects. Pregnant women usually prohibited from caring for dying person or attending funerals.

* **Home vs. hospital.** Dying in hospital may not be desirable for some patients who believe their spirit may get "lost" and not be able to find its way home. In addition, hospital environment may be seen as restrictive in meeting needs of extended family.

* **Special needs.** Some spiritual amulets, religious medallions, or rosary beads to be expected near patient. Prayers commonly practiced at bedside of dying patient. Roman Catholic faith provides for religious rite of Anointing of the Sick. If family's own priest unavailable, hospital chaplain or a member of health care team can perform this sacrament. Wailing is common and socially acceptable as sign of respect.

* **Care of the body.** Death very important spiritual event. Relative or member of extended family may help with the body. Family will request some time to say their good-byes before body is taken to morgue.

* **Attitudes toward organ donation.** Body extremely respected; majority of Catholics do not permit organ donation since body must be intact for burial.

* **Attitudes toward autopsy.** Same principle applies to autopsy. Becomes family matter, and must be decided by whole group.

Family Relationships

* **Composition/structure.** Mostly nuclear
families with extended family and
godparents (*compadres*). Familialism
dictates that family comes first. Help
first sought within immediate and
extended family. Strong sense of loyalty, reciprocity, and solidarity among
members. Behavior of individual
family members mediated by concern
for reputation of entire family.
Interpersonal relationships that are
nurturing, loving, intimate, and
respectful preferred. Gay and
lesbian relationships are not usually
acknowledged, but some families are
quite supportive.

    Traditionally, father or oldest male
is head of household and holds ultimate decision–making authority.
Deference to elders. Mothers, while
publicly deferential to husbands and
elders, hold great influence over their
children throughout lifespan; generally
respected for cultural wisdom and life
experience. Like all family members,
women expected to behave in manner
that maintains family's social
respectability. For this reason, Mexican
American women especially reluctant
to report domestic violence. Educated
and acculturated Mexican Americans
generally reflect more democratic
approach to family decision making.

    Respeto used to insure smooth
interpersonal relationships by demon-
strating respect for given individual.
Because of implied social power that
health care provider has as healer, failure to demonstrate *respeto* to Mexican
American clients could be perceived as
oppressive, classist, or racist.

    Respect for life, wisdom of elders,
family structure, hard work, bodily
integrity, and healthy living are some
cultural values that motivate many
people. Friendship and loyalty highly
valued, as are children and mothers.

* **Decision making.** Important decisions
may require consultation among
entire family.

* **Spokesperson.** Usually head of household.
Determine who is person of authority
and allow that person's input into decisions concerning care.

* **Gender issues.** *Machismo*, from word *macho*

(male), is complex cultural trait viewed stereotypically as brutish and controlling attitude toward women. Connotes "virile maleness" (which may emphasize bravery, honor, and integrity). Mexican American man expected to be strong, in control, and provider for family. Mexican American families commonly have democratic gender roles and shared decision making.

In contrast to stereotype of women as submissive and lacking in power and influence, mothers have considerable influence over family. Those who speak English acculturate more quickly than men, taking on more independent and multiple-role lifestyles typical of U.S. This can lead to role strain and gender conflict. Cost of living in U.S. necessitates dual family income, leading to more democratic and flexible male and female roles. *Chicana* feminist movement during 1960's and 1970s did much to discourage outright sexism.

Publicly, most women defer to husband and involve him in discussions surrounding plan of care. Lesbian women will generally extend this courtesy to their partners.

* **Caring role.** Women primary caregivers. Exceedingly stressful for individual to be separated from family group. Also psychologically difficult for family to hand over care of ill member to non-family health provider.

* **Expectations of and for children.** Children raised in protective environment. Expected to be obedient and respectful. Hard work and achievement encouraged; next generation is expected to "do better" than previous one. Children especially traumatized by separation from family members. Parents usually stay with child.

* **Expectations of and for elders.** Mexican American culture maintains reverence for elders; elders treated respectfully and in a formal manner. Elders actively involved in care and education of children. Avoid using first names when addressing elders.

* **Expectations of adults in caring for children and elders.** Women responsible for total support of children and elders. Patient teaching activities usually well

respect for authority and power of health care providers.

Curanderos. Attempt to correct imbalances by using prayers, pledges to religious or supernatural forces, and rituals involving candles, artifacts (such as eggs), herbal baths. Includes belief in humoral theory of disease. *Curandera,* or female folk healer, believed to be chosen by God to heal. Some of these individuals are listed in mental health agencies as "ethnopsychologist" or "ethnotherapist" in areas with large Mexican American populations.

Yerbalistas (Herbalists). Herbalism, dating from pre-Colombian times, plays key role in home remedies. Diagnoses made and herbal prescriptions brought home and made into broth or tea for patient to drink. Herbalism experiencing rebirth in U.S.

Sobadoras (masseuses). *Sobadoras* are female healers who use massage or manipulation of bones and joints to correct musculoskeletal imbalances. They are frequently also *parteras,* women who assist in pregnancy care and birth. Many *sobadoras* skilled in external rotation of fetus from breech to head down presentation.

As noted earlier, patients do not readily volunteer their belief in folk health system. Younger generations may have little belief in or knowledge of folk illnesses, remedies or healers. However, information can be obtained by talking and showing interest and acceptance of certain practices, such as use of herbs and teas. Herbal medicines can have powerful physiologic effects, some toxic. Many common herbs also have Spanish names. Often patient cannot identify herbal treatment by name.

There are also spiritual ceremonies for relief of symptoms and causative factors. One very common treatment for *mal de ojo* (evil eye) or *susto* (shock) is passage of unbroken raw egg over ill person, using sign of cross, candles, and associated prayer. Believed that illness will pass into egg and out of ill person's body.

Empacho (intestinal blockage) can be treated by massage of olive oil, warmed in spoon, then mixed with baking soda or powder in *sobradora's* hands. Patient lies down and is massaged front, then back. At end of massage, skin in center of back is pulled up until it makes a popping sound.

Combination of humoral and herbal medicine traditionally passed on from mother to daughter throughout successive generations. Continues to be used in U.S. by traditional Mexican Americans as alternative for minor medical, psychosocial, and chronic problems.

* **Acceptance of procedures.** During pregnancy, medications (including iron and vitamins) sometimes seen as potentially dangerous and avoided. Other women will take vitamins and iron during pregnancy, but cease taking them immediately after delivery, believing they will cause excessive weight gain.

  May believe reason for hospitalization is only to have particular symptom alleviated. "Doctors have that power" based on book learning and technology. Patients cooperative and supportive and will not interfere with hospital routine. Procedures usually accepted if practitioner trusted.

* **Care seeking.** Home care usually provided by female members of household. Many will not seek medical assistance until home remedies have failed and illness interferes with ability to meet role expectations. More acculturated individuals with adequate health insurance will seek medical assistance sooner. May believe illnesses not being treated unless medication prescribed. Specific diets should be discussed and could be emphasized as "prescriptions." Limited or lack of health care related to low financial resources, inadequate transportation, fear of legal authorities (in undocumented individuals), or perceived lack of *respeto*. Some Mexican Americans travel to Mexico for health care, probably related to need to be with extended family and distrust of U.S. health care practices.

Health Practices

* **Concept of health.** Health is feeling well and being able to maintain role function.
* **Health promotion and prevention.** Traditional Mexican Americans generally do not subscribe to usual health

maintenance and illness prevention strategies such as health screening or periodic check-ups, due to present-time orientation and belief that future is in God's hands. More acculturated or educated individuals demonstrate lifestyles more oriented to health promotion and disease prevention. Traditional Mexican American diet naturally nutritious and low in fat; however, introduction of fast food into diets of some immigrants has produced health risks. Alcohol consumption, smoking, and drug use more common among lower socioeconomic Mexican Americans born in U.S. than among those born in Mexico. Working women and teenagers report decreased quality of dietary intake.

* **Screening.** Mexican Americans will participate in medical screening if asked, providing rationale is explained. Because of modesty, many women delay Pap smears and mammograms, and are reluctant to perform breast self-examinations.

Selected References

Burk, M., Wieser, P., & Keegan, L. (1995). Cultural beliefs and health behaviors of pregnant Mexican-American women: Implications for primary care. *Advances in Nursing Science, 17*(4), 37-52.

Marin, G., & Marin, B. V. (1991). Research with Hispanic population. *Applied Social Research Methods Series, 23*, pp. 1–41. California: Sage Publications.

Meier, M., & Ribera, F. (1993). *Mexican Americans/ American Mexicans: From conquistadors to Chicanos.* New York: Hill and Wang.

Reinert, B. R. (1986). The health care beliefs and values of Mexican–Americans. *Home Healthcare Nurse, 4*(5), 23–31.

Authors

Tereza C. M. de Paula, RN, MS is a Clinical Nurse III at the Adult Medical Surgical Intensive Care Unit at the University of California, San Francisco Medical Center. She immigrated from Brazil to the United States in 1982 and established residence in San Francisco in 1987. Her field of interest is in the education of nursing staff to culturally diverse patient/families responses to hospitalization.

Kathleen Lagana, RN, PCNS, PhD is a specialist in low birthweight prevention and women's health. She travels extensively in Mexico and has done ethnographic field research on the Mexican American pregnancy experience. She received her PhD in Nursing at the University of California, San Francisco School of Nursing.

Leticia Gonzalez-Ramirez, RN, BS, works in primary and community health in the Salinas Valley in California and has done field research on Mexican American health issues. She received her BSN in nursing at University of San Francisco.

important than length. Negotiate time with client at beginning of interaction.

Rather than fatalistic, Puerto Ricans have a realistic, serene view of life. Some believe that destiny, or *Si Dios quiere* (If God wants), or spiritual forces are in control of life situations, health, and even death. As coping behavior, often used in times of crisis, death, or grief. Health and illness behaviors might be defined under this life perspective, influencing perception of future and control over life situations. Most Puerto Ricans open to discussing this view. Be clear and honest when assessing each individual's perceptions or view of life and how he/she perceives forces that control health and illness.

* **Consents.** Nonverbal communication plays vital role in acquiring informed consent for medical/surgical procedures, care of infant, research, and any other nursing/medical activity. In conversation, many will nod affirmatively but not necessarily mean agreement or understanding of dialogue or declaration. Using friendly and respectful approach, acceptable to ask for clarification/repetition of information provided. To avoid misunderstandings and legal consequences, health care professionals must provide an option for language preference for verbal or written information needed. Time also critical component for informed consent. Allow time for client to read and share decision with family members. Some would like to obtain verbal approval from another family or community member who is respected in health matters. When obtaining consent from a woman, consider obtaining verbal approval from partner. When feasible, verbal consent is preferable to signed approval.

* **Privacy.** Most Puerto Ricans open to expressing their physical ailments and discomforts to health care professionals. Private environment preferred for disclosure of health matters. Client often expects respectful environment with soft tone of voice when discussing these matters. More time might be needed for interview/assessment to be effective. Rooms without doors considered disrespectful

225

and conspicuous, especially if visits require removal of any clothing.

* **Serious or terminal illness.** Terminal illness often kept secret from patient. This protective mechanism, seldom discussed within family, allows family to ameliorate suffering of patient, provide optimistic atmosphere, and provide best quality of life for patient. Upon admission, ask patient (and document) name of family member ultimately responsible for patient's health decisions (i.e., self, oldest daughter/son, partner, caregiver).

Activities of Daily Living

* **Modesty.** Modesty highly valued among most men and women. Sexuality issues such as birth control, impotence, sexually transmitted disease, and infertility difficult to disclose. Generally, the word *sexo* (sex), is not used; instead, *tener relaciones* (to have intimate relations) is used. Preferably member of same gender should be present or assist with assessment. Men might use denial as coping strategy when discussing impotence. Most women prefer to meet and discuss health issues with provider before clothes are changed for breast, vaginal, or complete physical examinations. During hospitalization, men and women prefer to wear underwear and pants under hospital gowns.
* **Skin care.** Daily showers viewed as essential to promoting health and for personal appearance, except during illnesses such as colds, flu, or viral infection. Women may use rice or lemon water to wash their face. Women use roots of *maguey* (a medicinal plant) with epsom salts to prevent and treat acne.
* **Hair care.** Prefer to shampoo daily except for those women who avoid shampooing during menstruation. Some believe washing hair during menstruation or after giving birth may cause bleeding, stroke, abdominal pain, and arthritis. Not uncommon for women to use strong peroxide solutions with chamomile water in shampooing, believed to brighten and strengthen the hair.
* **Nail care.** No special beliefs.
* **Toileting.** During hospitalization, some may refrain from having bowel movement

expression as an exaggeration. Accept as socially learned mechanism to express and cope with pain. *Ay bendito!* is a verbal moaning expression of *dolor* (pain). Numerical scale to express pain might be difficult for rural elderly to understand. Prefer PO or IV medications for pain rather than IM or rectal. Herbal teas, heat, prayer used to manage pain.

* **Dyspnea.** *Asfixiado*—word describing shortness of breath. Fanning or blowing into patient believed to provide oxygen or relieve dyspnea. Tea from alligator's tail, snails, or *Savila* (plant leaf) believed to improve/heal dyspnea-related illnesses such as asthma and CHF.

* **Nausea/vomiting.** An alarming, recognized, but embarrassing symptom of illness. Many like to smell *alcoholado*—similar to isopropyl alcohol, or to apply it to the forehead to relieve nausea. Some put head between legs to stop vomiting. Mint, orange, or lemon tree leaves, or Star anise seeds boiled and used as tea to relieve nausea/ vomiting or stomach illnesses. Suppositories seldom used. Explain use of suppositories, since many believe they induce diarrhea.

* **Constipation/diarrhea.** Both seen as result of harmful food. Several natural and common laxatives such as milk of magnesia or castor oil used when people develop constipation. Hot prunes believed to relieve constipation. Many from rural areas frequently and inappropriately use enemas.

* **Fatigue.** Seen as a symptom of illness, anemia, malnutrition or *nervios* (nervousness). People who are under family or work stress may have *ataques de nervios* (nervousness attack).

* **Depression.** Suffering of *nervios* or *ataque de nervios*, rather than of depression is commonly described for symptoms related to depression. History of mental illnesses in patients or family members carries shame and stigma and might not be disclosed. Acknowledge confidentiality of any information provided.

* **Self-care for symptom management.** Natural herbal teas used for signs or symptoms of illness. Many consult family and

friends before consulting health care provider. Pharmacists often considered close community member of family, and play a vital role in symptom management.

Birth Rituals/Care of the New Mother/Baby

* **Pregnancy care.** Pregnancy a time of indulgence for women in many families. All favors and wishes granted for well-being of woman and baby. Men behave with tolerance, understanding, and patience at women's preferences. Diet followed carefully. Exercise viewed as inappropriate, and lifting objects prohibited. Rest and plenty of sleep recommended. Nurses should encourage regular exercise and good nutrition rather than too much eating.

  Many women choose to refrain from *tener relaciones* (sexual intercourse) during and after the second trimester. Men often see this time as opportunity for extramarital sexual activities. With caution and sensitivity, nurses may ask men about this issue and educate men about STD and AIDS risks resulting from multiple sexual partners.

* **Labor practices.** Hygiene and modesty highly respected during labor. Women prefer to have their body covered and not be examined frequently. Prefer bed position for labor. Prefer hospital environment with spouse or family member, mother or sister, present during labor.

* **Role of the laboring woman during birth process.** Active and demanding role assumed. Loud or noisy expressions of pain socially acceptable and encouraged to cope with pain and discomfort. Pain medications desirable. Explain to mother about pain management choices, risks, and benefits.

* **Role of the father and other family members during birth process.** Fathers assume passive, supportive role during labor. Young fathers prefer to attend birth classes to assist during labor. Others prefer not to be present during labor but wish to be informed frequently.

  Vaginal vs. cesarean section. Vaginal delivery preferred. For some, cesarean section carries "weak woman" stigma. Discuss options and choices early in pregnancy and educate patient about birth

authorization from several family members. Meeting and knowing organ recipient very important.

* **Attitudes toward autopsy.** Body is sacred and regarded with great respect. Autopsies usually seen as violation of body. Explain the need for autopsy with respect, soft tone of voice and in detail. Be sure to obtain verbal authorization from family leaders.

Family Relationships

* **Composition/structure.** Nuclear and extended family structure. All activities, decisions, social and cultural standards conceived around *la familia* (family). Many families still struggling with acceptance of homosexual behaviors. Sexual preferences usually undisclosed to avoid family rejection. Younger families more supportive and open to gay and lesbian family members.

* **Decision making.** Many Puerto Ricans still consult adults and elderly in decision-making issues as sign of respect and search for wisdom. Several family members might be involved in decision making. *Compadres* and *comadres* (godfather/godmother), still consulted in some families. In many families, oldest son/daughter in power positions to make final decision over health matters. In women's health related matters, husbands must be consulted to obtain verbal consent. If ignored, woman might be physically or emotionally harmed. Ask woman if husband must be consulted for authorization before signing for surgical or non-surgical procedures. Be aware that generational differences exist and some of above might not be true for young. Acceptable to ask and discuss with family about their decision-making plans.

* **Spokesperson.** Oldest daughter/son, older women in family. Husband in case of young children or women's issues.

* **Gender issues.** Older women might have po[w]erful and respected role in family. I[n] younger families, men expected t[o] responsibility in decision making[.]

* **Caring role.** Women assume active role [car]ing for ill. Men assume passive [role,] are to provide financially for [ill.] Because sick person is to ass[ume pas]sive role, this may hinder re[covery.]

could contradict Western medicine beliefs about self-care. Avoid confrontations with family. In hospitals, explain importance of self-care activities that lead to quick return home. This encourages cooperation with such activities as deep breathing and coughing, hygiene, ambulation.

* **Expectations of and for children.** Children are center of family life. Strong emphasis given to respect, education, and religion. In many homes, male children socialized in more independent macho role, while girls taught about home economics and family dynamics. Both negative and positive rewards used to encourage discipline, respect, and submission by children. Belts are used on legs or buttocks to physically discipline children. Mother usually assumes active role in discipline of children.

* **Expectations of and for elders.** *La abuela(o)* (grandparent or elderly) are figures of respect, admiration, and wisdom.

* **Expectations of adults in caring for children and elders.** Greatest role in caring for ill children placed on mother, with men assuming financial responsibilities. If mother must work outside home, great social and emotional burdens may develop. Assess for caregiver role overload or psychosocial stressors.

    Both men and women care for elderly. Responsibilities distributed and shared with family members and close network members. Family make noble financial and manpower efforts to keep elderly at home. Family members with higher social positions may take financial responsibility in exchange for efforts of those who cannot provide financially. Nursing homes or extended nursing care facilities seen as inappropriate and inconsiderate to elderly, and can lead to depression and distress among family members. Provide information, time to listen to concerns of different family members, and offer various choices. Best time-saving alternative is to coordinate time when all family members can be present to discuss discharge plans and issues in a conference-like environment.

Expectation of visitors. Neighbors, close and distant family members, and family

family members before consulting physician or nurse.

Health Practices

* **Concept of health.** *Llenitos y limpios*, not being too thin and being clean, are perceived as healthy. Health viewed as absence of mental, spiritual, or physical discomforts. "If you are happy, oversized, and have red cheeks, you are healthy." Someone who is worried or *nervioso(a)* is considered ill. Being underweight or thin is also seen as unhealthy and as symbol of economic disadvantage.

* **Health promotion and prevention.** Eating well and drinking fruit beverages are common health promotion practices. Multivitamins are commonly used to promote health and to prevent illnesses. Regular exercise needs to be stressed, because not perceived as health promotion practice and discouraged during an illness. Nurses should encourage and reinforce need for low fat/low cholesterol diet. Take advantage of every opportunity to teach about body weight and its influence on development of heart disease and other illnesses.

* **Screening.** Most men resistant to concept of health screening. Wives very influential in men's screening decisions. Women's breast and pelvic cancer screening procedures seen as intrusive and embarrassing and thus delayed or not done. Younger women more likely to participate in health screening activities. Elderly might be influenced by son/daughter to be screened and followed up for care. Health screening recommendations for children are well followed. Inform women about options and choices with breast and pelvic annual examinations. Female physicians preferred.

Selected References

Facundo, A. (1991). Sensitive mental health services for low-income Puerto Rican families. In M. Sotomayo (Ed.), *Empowering Hispanic families: A critical issue for '90s* (pp. 121-139). Milwaukee, WI: Family Service America.

García-Coll, C., & Mattei, M. L. (Eds.). (1989). *T psychosocial development of Puerto Rican women.* N York: Prager.

Guarnaccia, P.J., De La Cancela, V., & Carillo, E. (1989). The multiple meanings of ataque de nervios in the Latino community. *Medical Anthropology, 11*(1), 47-62.

Jorge, A. (1995). Mesa blanca: A Puerto Rican healing tradition. In L. L. Adler & B. R. Mukherji (Eds.), *Spirit versus scalpel: Traditional healing and modern psychotherapy* (pp. 109-120). Westport, CT: Bergin & Garvey/ Greenwood Publishing Group, Inc.

Author
Teresa Juarbe, RN, PhD is Assistant Professor at the School of Nursing at San Jose State University. She is currently studying the factors that influence the promotion of heart health in Latina women in the United States. She is a first generation Puerto Rican who immigrated to the U.S. in 1983.

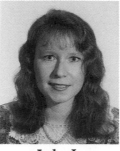

Luba J.
Evanikoff

Cultural/Ethnic Identity
* **Preferred term.** Russian.
* **History of immigration.** Major 20th Century Russian immigration occurred in five waves:

1900–1914　Mass of immigrants, primarily Christian Orthodox and Molokans (Christians who separated from Orthodox church in 18th century), fled Russia because of economic conditions, religious and political persecution.

1918–1940　Thousands of immigrants, mostly upper and middle class, army officers, and professionals, fearing for their lives, began to arrive as result of 1917 Bolshevik revolution.

1947–1952　About 20,000 immigrants, primarily war prisoners, slave laborers, or refugees from Germany during World War II arrived, refusing to return to Russia.

1971–1991　181,000 Russian Jews entered U.S. for religious and political reasons.

1988–present With rise of Gorbachev and beginning of breakup of U.S.S.R., thousands of immigrants, primarily Jewish, began to flee Russia.

* **Mape page.** *See Appendix C, p. 3 (top).*

Communication
* **Major language(s) and dialects.** Russian, a Slavic language with a Cyrillic alphabet, is major language in Russia with only a few dialectal differences. Major accents/dialects are southern, northern, and central. However, differences so minor that Russian-speaking person from north will understand southern dialect. Standard Russian language based on dialect of Moscow, which is primarily central and which contains

both southern and northern characteristics. Russian language very rich and expressive. Some of greatest literary works written in Russian, such as *War and Peace*, *Anna Karenina*, *Ruslan and Ludmilla*, and *Eugene Onegin*.

* **Literacy assessment.** Most recent immigrants highly educated and professionals (medical doctors, biomedical engineers, and engineers) and many are fluent in English. Recent immigrant patient may be health provider or have family member or friend who is one. English more of a problem among older immigrants.

* **Nonverbal communication.** Typically, direct eye-to-eye contact used. Russians very respectful to elders. Use touch freely with family and close friends. Personal space varies—close for friends/family; more distant until friendship or familiarity established. Nodding is gesture of approval.

* **Use of interpreters.** Because of language barrier, use interpreters whenever possible. Family and friends will get anxious when they have little information or understanding about diagnosis and prognosis of patient.

* **Greetings.** Taken very seriously. May shake hands or kiss each other on each cheek, depending on relationship. Elders highly respected and greeted with titles of "Mr." or "Mrs." or with "Uncle" and "Aunt" even in absence of blood relationship.

* **Tone of voice.** Sometimes loud, even in pleasant conversations.

* **Orientation toward time.** Most try to be on time for appointments and may even arrive early. Some older Jewish patients, having adapted to "working the system" in Soviet Russia for needed services, will either arrive early with frequent complaining or arrive late (those with less sense of urgency about their symptoms and to save time waiting), in order to guarantee being seen. These patients viewed as demanding and challenging.

* **Consents.** Explain procedures, tests, etc., with patient and family together. Most patients prefer to discuss with family members whether to sign consent form. Usually some family member

medical field and will offer further explanation and advice about consenting. Both patient and family will initiate appropriate questions to various procedures, tests, etc. Russians generally will not consent to be involved in research on experimental projects, procedures, or medications.

*   **Privacy.** Some patients prefer to have family member at bedside at all times. Others prefer some privacy.

*   **Serious or terminal illness.** In general, patients with terminal illnesses not told about their condition and prognosis. Family members need to be notified first. Then family will decide whether or not to tell patient. Usually, family members do not want patient to worry and be anxious about their terminal illness, adding another burden. Family wants patient to be at peace so physical and emotional condition does not worsen.

Activities of Daily Living

*   **Modesty.** Gender of provider not an issue. When doing peri-care or assessing urinary catheter, some patients prefer opposite gender family member to leave room. May not save urine for intake and output for reasons of modesty.

*   **Skin care.** When sick, some do not prefer daily showering; prefer sponge baths instead. See also Hair care.

*   **Hair care.** Hair washing not done as frequently when sick, especially when in hospital, for fear of catching cold or headache. If hair is to be washed, shut room windows and keep room warm, turning on heater if possible.

*   **Nail care.** Should be kept neatly trimmed.

*   **Toileting.** If bedridden, will not demand to use bathroom. Use of urinals, bedpans, and commodes accepted.

*   **Special clothing/amulet.** Some elderly women may prefer to wear warm clothing on top of hospital gowns for fear of catching cold or pneumonia. Some orthodox individuals may want to wear religious cross necklace. Allow use of religious medallions and pictures of saints.

*   **Self-care.** Hygiene may be performed by patient, family member, or with help of nurse or nurse's aide. Maintain modesty and privacy issues with

patient's opposite gender family member present.

Food Practices

* **Usual meal pattern.** Three meals a day, lunch the heaviest. Snacks in between with *chai* (hot tea) or fruit.
* **Special utensils.** Silverware.
* **Food beliefs and rituals.** When ill, prefer soft, warm or hot foods. Please see Food prescriptions.
* **Usual diet.** Russian food high in starch, fat, and salt. Please see Food prescriptions.
* **Fluids.** Hot tea - *chai* (chī), lukewarm drinks such as plenty of water, and fruit juices such as cranberry and apple. No ice in drinks! Label water pitcher "no ice."
* **Food prohibitions.** No pork or various shellfish with some Jewish and Molokan Russians. Need to inquire about other restrictions.
* **Food prescriptions.** When ill, prefer hot soups such as borscht, a vegetable, beet and cabbage soup; various light broth soups, such as chicken and rice soup; soft light (bland) foods such as oatmeal, ground meat patties, boiled chicken, baked and mashed potatoes, fresh fruit, vegetables, and plain yogurt. Drinks include *chai*, *chai* with lemon and honey or with various jams such as raspberry, strawberry, and lemon. Also hot milk with honey.

Symptom Management

* **Pain.** *Bohl-yeet* (pain) High pain threshold. Very stoic and may not ask for pain medications. Encourage pain medications as appropriate. Avoid offering morphine sulphate for fear of developing pneumonia and for fear of addiction. Will understand numerical scale of measuring pain.
* **Dyspnea.** *Odishka* (dyspnea) May get anxious because of language barrier. Will accept oxygen.
* **Nausea/vomiting.** *Toshnata* (nausea) Will accept nonpharmacological methods first. Offer lemon slices, ginger ale, mineral water, plain yogurt, and tea with lemon. May refuse to take routine medications when nauseated. Some nausea associated with taking too many medications, especially on empty stomach. (Some believe ingesting too many medications will poison body.)

Most medications should be taken with snacks, such as crackers, etc.

* **Constipation/diarrhea.** Regular bowel movements a priority. Offer prune juice and laxatives such as Milk of Magnesia or other laxatives of choice. Patient may refuse various procedures if "not feeling too well," nauseated, or constipated. Enemas widely accepted as general procedure for constipation. Will accept meds for diarrhea.

* **Fatigue.** *Ystalost* (fatigue) Rest and sleep best prescription. Some may accept or refuse sleeping pills for insomnia. Russians consider good night's sleep essential, and some will be upset if procedures require disturbing their sleep. Explain need before bedtime.

* **Depression.** *De-pre-si-a* (depression) Most Russians do not like to take excessive medications. Discuss with patient and family. Spend time with patient to show that patient is cared for.

* **Self-care for symptom management.** Usually relies on self-care first before seeking medical attention. See Home and folk remedies.

Birth Rituals/Care of the New Mother/Baby

* **Pregnancy care.** With some patients, prenatal care not expected unless pregnant mother feels something is wrong. Pregnant women protected from bad news, believed potentially harmful to fetus. Pregnant mother can work outside home until last trimester. During whole course of pregnancy, mother discouraged from lifting any heavy objects or from skipping any steps when climbing or going down stairs, for fear of losing fetus. During last trimester, mother especially discouraged from lifting any objects, such as chairs or boxes. Also discouraged from performing heavy exercise, such as jumping or jogging. Believed that these activities may harm fetus: umbilical cord may become wrapped around baby and the baby may choke or baby may move to breech position or become past due.

* **Labor practices.** When pregnant mother senses time of delivery is near, she is encouraged to drink castor oil (although practice slowly fading) or is given an enema for easier birth. If M.D. not available, then midwife can assist with delivery. Mother highly

encouraged to walk when contractions begin, to promote dilatation. During traditional births, mother discouraged from taking any pain medication during labor for fear of harm to baby or herself (e.g., epidurals), but some may want it. Stimulation and lighting in birthing room should be minimal. Believed that newborn's eyes are not yet strong or mature enough, and too much light will cause baby to develop poor eyesight.

* **Role of the laboring woman during birth process.** Russian women generally assume passive role during birthing process; follow commands of doctor or midwife. Depending on individual, Russian mothers generally are not very loud when giving birth.

* **Role of the father and other family members during birth process.** Traditionally, father plays passive role; is not allowed in birthing room. Only closest female family member allowed, such as maternal mother, sister, or mother-in-law (whoever is available at time), but may vary, depending on level of acculturation.

* **Vaginal vs. cesarean section.** Vaginal delivery highly preferred over cesarean. In Russia, if baby in breech position, all possible measures taken by physician to ensure vaginal delivery.

* **Breastfeeding.** Breastfeeding an expectation of all Russian mothers until milk "runs out" (even to toddler years). Russian mothers know importance of breastfeeding, such as health benefits and immunological properties that can be passed to baby. Russian mothers' partners support and encourage breastfeeding. In Russia, even societal support for breastfeeding is given. Employers provide child care at work site, and average maternity leave is about 25 months. Important for breastfeeding mother to be at peace. Believed that baby may become "hyper" later in life if there is too much noise or stimulation or if mother is nervous when breastfeeding. If breastfeeding mother suddenly shocked or scared for any reason, first breast milk should be expelled before feeding baby again. This milk considered unhealthy, and may cause baby to develop diarrhea. Russian mothers

breastfeed in dim light to save baby's eyesight. When breastfeeding, breasts should be kept warm at all times, such as dressing warmly; believed to prevent mother from developing breast cancer later in life.

* **Birth recuperation.** Traditional practices are 15 days of bedrest. Cooking and other various household chores done by mother's mother or other appropriate person for up to 40 days. During these 40 days, new mother should remain at home and not go outside. Believed that new mother's internal organs should heal and return to their pre-pregnant position during birth recuperation to prevent future physical problems. Traditionally, new mother wears pelvic binder to regain her figure. Peri-care with warm water important.

* **Problems with baby.** If problem with baby, first notify mother of baby; she may not want anyone else to know.

    Important to keep baby warm at all times to keep baby's bones developing normally and to prevent illnesses. Baby's head should always be covered when exposed to cold, wind, or very hot sun.

* **Male and female circumcision.** In general, Russian Christian parents do not believe in male circumcision. Some Jewish parents prefer male circumcision. Discuss with parents. Female circumcision never performed.

Death Rituals

* **Preparation.** Inform head of family first; he/she may not want patient to know to ensure a peaceful death. Ask family about notifying rabbi, priest, or minister. In general, some family members may decide that elderly patient should be DNR (Do Not Resusite) to die in comfort rather than on life support.

* **Home vs. hospital.** If patient terminally ill, family will prefer to have patient live at home and be taken care of by all family members. In general, Russians do not favor nursing homes and related health care facilities. If patient placed in such a facility, should be near family members' home. Russians may be selective about choosing health care facility for their loved ones. If patient acutely ill, family will prefer patient to stay in hospital.

* **Special needs.** May need rabbi, priest, minister, or other individuals to pray for patient. Discuss with family.
* **Care of the body.** Depending on religion, family members may want to wash the body and put special clothing on the deceased. Some Jewish persons believe that body should remain intact; thus, severed limbs should be placed back on the body if possible. Most Russian Christians do not believe in cremation. Discuss with family.
* **Attitudes toward organ donation.** In general, most Russians believe that body is sacred and thus do not believe in organ donation.
* **Attitudes toward autopsy.** Body is respected and considered sacred. Unless absolutely necessary, most Russians will refuse autopsy.

Family Relationships

* **Composition/structure.** Extended family with strong family bonds and great respect for elders. Family-oriented. Gays and lesbians are not acknowledged.
* **Decision making.** Father, mother, eldest son, or eldest daughter.
* **Spokesperson.** Same as above or strongest personality.
* **Gender issues.** No major gender issues. Although husband and wife will consult with each other, some wives may eventually give way to husband's opinion. The more dominant personality will probably prevail.
* **Caring role.** Whole family pulls together during crisis for support and strength.
* **Expectations of and for children.** Children taught to behave, be obedient, be very respectful to elders, to study hard and obtain a higher education. Children also expected to take turns caring for ill family members.
* **Expectations of and for elders.** Elders highly respected and expected to also care for ill if possible. Elders live in extended families, are family-oriented, and expect their children also to be family-oriented and to produce offspring. Elders also expected to rear their grandchildren, especially when parents work.
* **Expectations of adults in caring for children and elders.** Adults expected to care for ill family members and accept their parents into home to be cared for.

* **Expectation of visitors.** Family members and friends expected to visit sick at hospital. Russians have strong bonds and provide strength and support for sick. Give quick orientation of hospital unit, such as location of pantry (if appropriate), linen closet, and cafeteria.

Spiritual/Religious Orientation

* **Primary religious/spiritual affiliation.** Predominantly Jewish and Eastern Orthodox. Other religions include Molokans, Seventh Day Adventists, Pentecostals, Old Believers, and Baptists.
* **Usual religious/spiritual practices.** Because of prohibition of religion in former U.S.S.R., most recent immigrants may not practice religion. However, some individuals who are Jewish, Eastern Orthodox, or Protestant will pray in their own way.
* **Use of spiritual healing/healers.** Nurse needs to allow for rabbi, priest, or minister to visit and pray for patient. Discuss with patient and family.

Illness Beliefs

* **Causes of physical illness.** Poor nutrition, not dressing warmly, family history, stress, and pregnant mother not taking care of herself or ingesting too many medications. Some Christian faiths believe illness is "will of God," "God's punishment," or "test of one's faith in God."
* **Causes of mental illness.** Stress and moving into new environment.
* **Causes of genetic defects.** See Causes of physical illness.
* **Sick role.** Ill family member always taken care of by family. May even bring nutritious and appropriate food from home. In general, ill patients place themselves on bed rest. Explain importance of ambulation and other practices, such as use of incentive spirometer.
* **Home and folk remedies.** Russians will treat themselves first before seeking medical attention and believe that excessive drug use can be harmful and that all drugs are poison in some way. Home and folk remedies include rubbing of camphor ointment and other various mixtures, oils, and ointments, placement of hot glasses on bare back (very old fashioned treatment),

enemas, light exercise with fresh air and some sunlight, mud baths, steam baths, mineral water, sweet liquor, herbal teas, tea with lemon, honey, and jam, and hot soups.

* **Acceptance of procedures.** Please see Consents. Most Russians may refuse blood transfusions for fear of contracting HIV/AIDS. Unfamiliarity with routines and equipment may cause problems in care. Orient Russian patients thoroughly to routines and explain equipment (i.e., changing IV heparin locks every three days, how and why intake and output are measured, and "alarm" feature of IV equipment). Russian patient may lay awake all night in fear that their IV tubing will develop "air in the line" by the bag running dry, not knowing that the IV pump would alarm. Some diabetic patients may resist new regime because they have treated themselves for years.
* **Care seeking.** Some Russians may seek medical care as last resort. Home and folk remedies tried first. See Home and folk remedies.

Health Practices

* **Concept of health.** Regular bowel movements, absence of symptoms such as colds.
* **Health promotion and prevention.** Good health maintained by dressing warmly, eating nutritious foods, having regular bowel movements, and exercising, such as walking in open air with some sunshine, and pleasant entertainment. In addition, if patient has fever and/or is diaphoretic, highly important to keep patient covered (not necessarily with heavy blanket) and to shut window. Russians believe they are most prone to catching pneumonia at this time. Staying warm, dressing warmly, and avoiding ice cold drinks when ill emphasized in health promotion and prevention.
* **Screening.** Russians respect medical doctors and will disclose pertinent information. Russians often mistake registered nurses in U.S. for medical doctors because of RN's professional role. Will not usually go for screening procedure (i.e., mammogram) unless person feels something is wrong.

Selected References

Bonfante, G. (1982). Russian. In W.D. Halsey & E. Friedman (Eds.), *Collier's encyclopedia*, 20, p. 295. New York: Macmillan.

Brod, M. (1992). Older Russian emigrès and medical care. *Western Journal of Medicine*, *157*, 333-336.

Miner, J., Witte, D. J., & Nordstrom, D. L. (1994). Infant feeding practices in a Russian and a United States city: Patterns and comparisons. *Journal of Human Lactation*, 10(2), 95-97.

Werstman, V. (1977). *The Russians in America: A chronology fact book 1727-1970*, 24, pp. 8-19. New York: Oceana Publications.

Wheat, M. E., Brownstein, H., & Kritash, V. (1983). Aspects of medical care of Soviet Jewish emigrès. *Western Journal of Medicine*, 139, 900-904.

Author

Luba J. Evanikoff, RN, BSHS, BSN is a Clinical Nurse II at the University of California, San Francisco Medical Center in the Cardiology Telemetry and Cardiovascular and Cardiothoracic Surgery Units. Immigrating from Russia in 1947 and 1958, Luba's parents met, married, and raised Luba in the United States. She is grateful that they have encouraged and guided her in preserving her Russian culture.

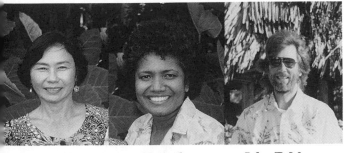

*Dianne N.
Ishida*

*Tusitala
Feagaiga
Toomata-Mayer*

John F. Mayer

Cultural/Ethnic Identity

*   **Preferred terms.** Samoan, Western Samoan
(*Samoa i Sisifo*), American Samoan
(*Amerika Samoa*). Politically there are
two Samoas: Western Samoa, an inde-
pendent nation with historically strong
British ties, and American Samoa, a
U.S. territory. They share a common
language and culture.

*   **History of immigration/migration.**

1920s   Small scale immigration to U.S.,
mostly through religious affiliations. (The La'ie Samoan
community in Hawaii dates to
1920s and is oriented to Latter
Day Saints church.)

1951   U.S. Naval Base in American
Samoa closed when administra-
tion of Territory transferred to
U.S. Department of the Interior.
Approximately 2,000 American
Samoan government workers and
their dependents immigrated to
Hawaii and California by 1952.

1970s   Downturn in New Zealand economy in 1970s caused many Western
Samoans to immigrate to
American Samoa and then to
U.S. Travel facilitated by improve-
ments to international airport in
Western Samoa in the 1980s and
increased airline services to both
Samoas. Unlike previous waves,
many later immigrants had less
education and fewer marketable
job skills.

*   **Map page.** (Please note that Swains Island,
also called *Olohenga* and geographically
part of the *Tokelau* Group, is
politically part of the unincorporated
territory of American Samoa.)
See Appendix C, p. 4.

Communication

* **Major language(s) and dialects.** Samoan is official language of both Samoas. No significant dialectal variation throughout both Samoas. English is language of instruction in schools after early grades. Both Samoan and English used in government communications, business, and mass media, although Samoan preferred.

* **Literacy assessment**. Until recently, virtually universal secular-based literacy instruction (village pastor's school) conducted throughout both Samoas. Thus, most adults literate in Samoan and speak English to some degree. Because of recent increased levels of educational attainment, young adults of the 1990s have greater proficiency in English than their parents or grandparents. Young Samoans often act as interpreters for older family members. Because of dialectal variation in English (New Zealand English in Western Samoa vs. American English in American Samoa), Western Samoans may not be familiar with American terminology or local idioms. Use simple medical terms.

* **Nonverbal communication.** Samoan society stresses politeness and deference to those in perceived positions of authority (e.g., clergy, family chief or *matai* [mah tie], elderly, professionals). This often takes form of silence, agreement, or attempted compliance to requests or orders, whether or not fully understood. Physical space important, especially for adults. Area in front of person considered most important. Touching accepted as sign of sincerity or intimacy (e.g., on the shoulder, clasping hands). When speaking before a group, eye contact generally avoided. During personal conversation, eye contact may vary, depending on circumstances. Appropriate in casual or informal exchanges, except in situations of wide social distance. Relative height important in Samoan society. Customary for inferiors to maintain a lower posture (e.g., sitting down) than superiors, although prolonged exposure to New Zealand and American customs may cause individuals to reverse this relationship. Question and

answer format of conversation among adults more appropriate for intimate conversation in Samoa. In formal situations (e.g., conferences), customary to expect complete presentation by health care provider to be answered by similar presentation from family spokesperson. Custom requires both polite and honorific speech as well as Christian and biblical references.

* **Use of interpreters.** Decisions involve all adults within family or 'aiga (ah ing ah); therefore, families may want to include more than immediate family members in conferences. Customary for single spokesperson to represent family and voice decisions, usually the family head (matai) or older relative. Individual acting as spokesperson may vary; both women and men may take this role. Younger family members more proficient in English may serve as interpreters. Non-family members may also serve as interpreters, especially ministers of any denomination and professional people (e.g., social workers, police, teachers). Male and female members of same family (related by blood) will avoid conversations focusing on sexual issues, a deep feature of Samoan culture, now fading among Samoans living abroad.

* **Greetings.** First names preferred. Sufficient exposure to Western culture created understanding and acceptance of use of last names. Handshake customary method of greeting for both males and females, also used when taking leave. Kissing restricted to instances of extreme emotion, although increased tendency for Samoans living in Hawaii to greet members of opposite sex with kiss (Hawaiian custom). Elderly may greet through touching noses, a practice becoming obsolete. Smiles can indicate happiness and contentment as well as defensive expression of unease or uncertainty. Raised eyebrows may be used informally to indicate affirmative response.

* **Tone of voice.** Because of open and communal nature of Samoan society, loud or disruptive levels of sound considered inappropriate. Conversation with family should be restricted to levels within hearing of family members only. Because of high value placed upon

Increasingly common, however, for modern Samoans to consume three meals a day. Fairly large portions are eaten, consisting of starch (taro, bananas, rice, or breadfruit) and some kind of meat protein. Although fish highly favored as protein source, modern Samoan diet leans heavily toward foods high in cholesterol and saturated fats. If no dietary restrictions prescribed, suggest that family bring in food prepared to patient's liking.

* **Food beliefs and rituals.** Traditional custom requires adults to eat before older children. In more acculturated families, all family members may eat together, although former practice may be preferred in presence of guests. Hot prepared meals preferred. Prayer may be said before every meal, especially dinner. Some prefer to eat with fingers.

* **Usual diet.** Starch such as taro, bananas, and breadfruit preferred. Rice and potatoes can be substituted. These starches eaten with beef, fish, pork, chicken, or canned meats. Sometimes combination of two or three meats eaten during one meal.

* **Fluids.** Frequent cool water or sweet drinks preferred if available. Tea or coffee often consumed with evening meals. Carbonated drinks highly favored form of fluid intake.

* **Food prohibitions.** Pregnant and postpartum women may have food restrictions.

* **Food prescriptions.** Warm soups and starches made with coconut cream preferred. Fish soups or soups made of very basic ingredients such as rice, onions, a few vegetables, and meats seasoned with salt and pepper or curry generally given to sick person. Sweet soups made of papaya or young coconut meat generally given to children or postpartum women. Fish soup preferred meal for sick person. Can be served with or without adding coconut cream.

Symptom Management

* **Pain.** *Tiga* (Tee ngah). May be stoic and non-complaining. Pain often accepted as God's will. Degree and type of pain may be hard for some patients to verbalize. Nurse may need to offer pain medications. Narcotic pain medications of any kind are

acceptable. Massage often used traditionally for pain.

* **Dyspnea.** *Faigata le manava* (Faye gah tah leh mah nah vah)–trouble with breathing. Oxygen can be given after explanation of procedure. Shortness of breath may cause anxiety.

* **Nausea/Vomiting.** *Fa'afaufau* (fah ah fow)/ *fa'asuati* (fah ah soo ah tee). During periods of nausea, patient may want to rest. In pregnancy, nausea attributed to reaction to food. Traditional herbal medicine (both internal and external) addresses nausea.

* **Constipation/Diarrhea.** *Manava mamau* (mah nah vah mah oo)/*manava tata* (mah nah vah tuh taahh). Sometimes attributed to what one ate and should not have eaten. Gastrointestinal ailments categorized as those causing constipation, diarrhea, or pain. Patients embarrassed to talk about feces. Nutritional controls acceptable for constipation and diarrhea. Use enemas as last resort.

* **Fatigue.** *Vaivai* (vie)—weak. Fatigue caused from overexertion, heat, or illness. Because Samoans traditionally tend to be early risers, afternoon napping not uncommon.

* **Depression.** Depression, especially of a relative, signal for increased interpersonal interaction within family. Patient is focus of physical, emotional, and psychological interaction. May be a tendency to somatize general complaints.

* **Self-care for symptom management.** Samoans tend to avoid self-treatment even if minor. Other family members become involved. Traditional healer may be consulted by family for assessment and treatment with Samoan medicine. Continued care undertaken by family as a whole.

Birth Rituals/Care of the New Mother/Baby

* **Pregnancy care.** Pregnancy (*Ma'itaga* [mah ee tah ngah], *ma'ito* [mah ee toe]) considered an illness. Prenatal care may vary tremendously and may involve early traditional practices or Western-oriented care. Many Samoans may not be familiar with availability and scope of Western prenatal care. Pregnant women cannot eat certain foods such as octopus or raw fish and cannot eat alone or be left unattended, especially at night. Pregnancy prohibitions

* **Spokesperson.** In interactions with non-Samoans, family chief, elder, or most educated family member (if English a problem) may serve as spokesperson.
* **Gender issues.** Family members traditionally had gender specific roles, often adaptable, depending on circumstances. Men performed heavier outdoor activities (e.g., fishing, building, and preparing the earth oven) and took part in village council. Women and children performed tasks necessary for maintenance of household (e.g., child care, weaving). Both males and females took part in agricultural activities and some food preparation.
* **Caring role.** Women are primary bedside caregivers, but children may assist. Female-male blood relatives have a gender avoidance taboo which may affect selection of a caregiver.
* **Expectations of and for children.** Children valued, even if out of wedlock, but are expected to be obedient, serve older family members, and avoid direct confrontation with those in authority. Parents indulgent with very young children. Older children generally responsible for care of younger siblings and expected to have high degree of autonomy at early age. Peers play major role in socialization.
* **Expectations of and for elders.** Elders are traditionally revered as sources of wisdom and knowledge of the Samoan way, or *Fa'a-Samoa* (fah ah sah mo ah), and continue to be active part of family. Often assist in child care, decision making, and oversee family activities.
* **Expectations of adults in caring for children and elders.** Multiple parenting, with aunts, grandparents, and older children sharing responsibility for childrearing. After weaning, younger children become responsibility of older children. Children also may be assigned to care for an elder. Samoan society instills life-long sense of duty to care for parents that may override marital and social responsibilities.
* **Expectation of visitors.** Reception of guests in Samoan society institutionalized through formal rituals and daily practices. Food exchange important. Visitors can expect high degree of formality, especially during initial visits. Visitors should first approach

eldest adult to show respect. Visitors generally welcomed. (See Nonverbal communication). In hospital, family member may intercede with visitors on behalf of patient.

Spiritual/Religious Orientation

*   **Primary religious/spiritual affiliation.** Since introduction of Christianity in 1830, both American and Western Samoa virtually 100% Christian. Most common denominations: Congregational, Methodist, Catholic, Latter Day Saints, Seventh Day Adventist, Assembly of God. Baha'i faith also enjoys some following in Western Samoa. Modern Samoan oratory (chiefly speech) and formal speech may be used during family crises and incorporates many biblical and Christian references.

*   **Usual religious/spiritual practices.** Christian prayer conducted before all group interactions or family gatherings. Christian religion forms major foundation of all Samoan social intercourse. Therefore, some form of group prayer led by the family spokesperson precedes and concludes all such interaction. Minister occupies highest rung of Samoan social ladder. Communal nature of Samoan society requires visits to hospital by religious sub-groups from within religious community or church to which patient belongs; may include church choir, women's group, church youth group, and high ranking church-community officials. Specific practices depend upon religious denomination (e.g., Congregational, Methodist, Catholic, Latter Day Saints, Seventh Day Adventist, Assembly of God, Pentecostal, etc.).

*   **Use of spiritual healers.** Western medicine often used in conjunction with traditional Samoan medicine, based on herbal lore, physical manipulation and massage, and spiritual harmony. Traditional medicine usually confined to illnesses recognized as intrinsically 'Samoan' (indigenous maladies), or illnesses that have as their root cause, social or spiritual imbalance. Vagueness of these classifications may result in overlapping territoriality. Health care provider should be aware

of tendency of family members to rely upon Samoan medicine in event of uncertain prognoses or ineffective treatment by Western medicine.

Illness Beliefs

* **Causes of physical illness.** Illnesses categorized as those whose causes are apparent (such as trauma), those from the effects of internal/external ecosystem (such as parasites, diabetes, climate), those caused by germs, and those arising from supernatural causes (physical illness may sometimes be attributed to past misdeeds or conduct). Consequently, need for openness, trust, and harmony in healing process may require group confessions of past misdeeds. General malaise may be attributed to displaced life force, or *to'ala* (toe ah lah), in which therapeutic massage by healer can reinstate it to its proper location. Generally, illness disrupts normal order of family life. For this reason, Samoans tend to put off treatment until advanced illness requiring hospitalization. Samoan health beliefs and practices have expanded to incorporate Western beliefs and practices. Samoans believe that illnesses may be of European origin, *ma'i palagi* (mah ee pah lang ee), or Samoan origin, *ma'i samoa* (mah ee sah moa ah), and most effectively treated by those familiar with them. Thus, Western and Samoan medicine not seen as competing systems, but as complementary ones.

* **Causes of mental illness.** Mental illness may be caused by spirit possessions, stress from interpersonal relationships, family obligations, social constraints, and pressure from peer groups. Mental illness may also be attributed to guilt reaction from prior misdeeds.

* **Causes of genetic defects.** Genetic defects often considered punishment for bad behavior of husband during pregnancy, deviant or unacceptable behavior of pregnant mother or family member toward others, or violation of dietary taboos.

* **Sick role.** Sick are cared for and treated well by all family members.

* **Home and folk remedies.** Folk remedies (e.g., *fofo* [fuh foe] or massage and herbs) prevalent, especially in case of

261

illnesses attributed to Samoan causes. Patients may not readily admit to use of folk remedies.

* **Acceptance of procedures.** Blood transfusions may be acceptable if necessary for patient's survival.
* **Care seeking.** Except in cases of severe trauma and diseases clearly associated with Western origin, Samoans will usually seek aid of traditional healer before seeking care from Western doctors. Both Western and traditional services may be used at same time.

Health Practices

* **Concept of health.** *Soifua maloloina* (so ee fooah mah low low ee nah)—to live, rest, recover from sickness. Traditional view of health incorporates holistic approach, including aspects related to body or *fa'aletino* (fah ah lay tea no), mind or *fa'alemafaufau* (fah ah lay mah fow), and spirit or *fa'aleagaga* (fah ah lay ah ngah). Thus, concept of health attuned not only to obvious physical ailments (e.g., a broken leg), but also to individual's relationships with others (especially family), environment, and spiritual world (especially recently deceased ancestors). Illness therefore may be seen as consequence of one's actions toward living or dead, as well as violation of social or religious principles shared by society. Imbalances in physical-spiritual-mental harmony of individual require similarly holistic approach to healing process. Thus, treatment for illnesses in Samoan world may involve both Samoan and non-Samoan cures with no perception of conflicts between the two health systems.
* **Health promotion and prevention.** Ill health considered a problem when it begins to interfere with individual's ability to participate in day-to-day activities of family and social life. Concept of preventive health not well established in Samoa. Treatment (e.g., medication) often discontinued after symptoms abate since social and family participation again possible, and because continued attention given to illness may prolong distraction from full group participation.
* **Screening.** Great respect for authority means that screening by those in authority

(elders or the pastor) will pose no problem. Questions about sexually transmitted diseases, mental aberrations, sexual relations, menstrual cycle, feces, or genitalia may be considered shameful and private. Relevancy of questions must be clear. Samoans may find it difficult to undress for health care provider of opposite sex.

Selected References

King, A. P. (1990). A Samoan perspective: Funeral practices, death, and dying. In J. K. Parry (Ed.), *Social work practice with the terminally ill: A transcultural perspective* (pp. 175-189). Springfield, IL: Charles C. Thomas, Publisher.

Kinloch, P. (1985). *Talking health but doing sickness: Studies in Samoan health*. Wellington, New Zealand: Victoria University Press.

Macpherson, C., & Macpherson, L. (1990). *Samoan medical belief and practice*. Auckland: Auckland University Press.

Authors

Dianne Ishida, PhD, RN is an Assistant Professor at the School of Nursing at the University of Hawaii at Manoa. She is a nurse anthropologist whose focus is learning and culture (Pacific/Asian cultures) particularly Samoa.

Tusitala Toomata-Mayer, AS, RN is a registered nurse of Samoan background specializing in medical oncology at the Queen's Medical Center in Honolulu. She is also an international flight attendant with United Airlines and is currently completing her baccalaureate in nursing at the University of Hawaii at Manoa.

John F. Mayer, MA, PhD(c) is the Coordinator of the Samoan Language and Culture Program at the University of Hawaii at Manoa and a doctoral student in Applied Linguistics at the University of Hawaii.

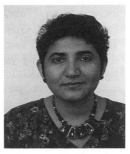

Rozina Rajwani

South Asians living in North America are heterogeneous in language and culture, and include those from India, Pakistan, Bangladesh, Sri Lanka, Nepal, as well as those from Fiji and East Africa whose origins are Indian Subcontinent. This chapter highlights three cultural groups: Hindus, Muslims, and Sikhs. Variations among South Asians also due to country of origin, level of education, social class, religious affiliation, background (rural or urban), and number of years lived in North America.

Cultural/Ethnic Identity
* **Preferred terms.** South Asians, East Indians, Asian Indians, or IndoAmericans. Sometimes identified by religious affiliations such as Sikhs, Hindus, Muslims, etc.
* **History of immigration.**

1901–1923	Over 6,000 East Indians, mostly Sikhs from Punjab, immigrated to U.S.
1923	Legislation prohibited further immigration. Between 1920-1930, 3,000 East Indians left America due to lack of work opportunities.
1946	1,500 East Indians remained in U.S. Legislation gave Asian Indians right to become American citizens and bring relatives to America (annual quota = 100).
1965	Revisions in U.S. immigration laws opened doors for highly educated, technically trained individuals to enter U.S. By 1985, South Asians numbered 526,223.
1987	Immigration Act of 1987 made visas easier to obtain. More than 20,000 East Indians migrating to U.S. each year.

* **Map page.** *See Appendix C, p. 1.*

Communication
* **Major language and dialects.** Common

Activities of Daily Living

* **Modesty.** Men comfortable with pajama top and bottoms; however, women prefer not to wear hospital clothes as body parts likely to show through. Hindu women may prefer to wear sari. Most Sikh and Muslim women prefer to wear *shalwar* (loose pants) and *kamiz* (top that is below knee length). Many would prefer to cover head and chest with rectangular cloth (*chader*, approximately 6' x 3').

* **Skin care.** Most South Asians like to take daily morning shower. Person with respiratory tract infection or prior surgery would prefer bed bath. They use a lot of running water when bathing as water considered symbol of purity.

* **Hair care.** Among many South Asian women, long hair considered sign of feminine beauty. Hair washed once or twice weekly. Women massage scalp with coconut or mustard oil weekly, and comb and braid hair daily. Usually wear head covering. Traditional Sikh male not supposed to cut their hair or shave their beard. Their hair usually secured in turban. No restrictions on cutting or shaving body hair among Hindus and Muslims.

* **Nail care.** Nails cut short and kept clean. No cutting of nails at night and once clipped, nail parings must be thrown in sink with running water.

* **Toileting.** South Asians prefer private toilets for elimination; however, also accept bedpans, urinals, or bedside commodes. Would like thorough peri-wash with water after elimination. Provide pint sized plastic water pitcher near commode for peri-care. They must use left hand to wash and wipe their perineal area. Muslims do not eliminate at certain times of day [e.g., at time of *Azan* (prayer) in mosque]. Strict Muslims must purify themselves by washing before prayer. No special rituals for elimination among Hindus and Sikhs.

* **Special clothing/amulets.** High caste Hindu men have a sacred thread tied around the body. Thread must never be removed without permission of patient or family member. Baptized Sikh men and women wear *kirpan* (a piece of cloth around chest), *Kanga* (a wooden

267

comb), *Kara* (an iron bracelet). *Kirpan*, *kara*, and *kanga* must never be removed. Muslims sometimes wear *Taawiz* (Koranic verses folded in small cloth) for protection, usually provided by high level spiritual person.

* **Self-care.** Sick individuals assume dependent sick role and expect caregiver or a family member to assist with personal hygiene and meals. Other family members relieve patient from family responsibilities to ensure physical and emotional rest.

Food Practices

* **Usual meal pattern.** South Asians usually eat two to three meals per day. Prefer big meal at lunch and small meal at supper. May prefer supper in late evening. During acute illness, may like bland, easily digested foods.

* **Special utensils.** Hindus may prefer to use metal utensils such as copper, brass, and iron for cooking and for eating as these considered sacred. Sikhs and Muslims have no such preferences in utensils.

* **Food beliefs and rituals.** Food given much respect in most South Asian religions. Advised that one must eat food with love and compassion and be thankful to God for giving food that alleviates hunger and nourishes body and mind. One must also avoid any form of distraction such as watching television, reading, or excessive talking while eating. Many South Asians use fingers of right hand to eat food and most prefer to wash their hands before touching food. Overeating discouraged equally in Hindu, Sikh, and Islam religions; believed that overeating decreases one's life span.

* **Usual diet.** Most common staple foods among Hindus, Sikhs, and Muslims are rice or *chapatti* (flat baked bread made with whole wheat flour) with meat, vegetable, or lentil curry. Sweet dishes not part of regular meal.

* **Fluids.** Instead of fruit juices or sodas, water or buttermilk (*lasi*) are beverages of choice; believed to help digestive processes. Tea is common hot beverage instead of coffee.

* **Food prohibitions**.
    Hindus: refrain from eating any kind of meat and fish. Some may not

even eat eggs. Alcohol permitted only in moderation. Foods may not be eaten during observance of fast. May fast one day each week or each month; may be total abstinence of food and fluid or eating foods that are pure (for example, fruit, yogurt, and nuts).

Muslims: observe fast during month of *Ramazan* (a Muslim calendar month). No food and fluids allowed from sunrise to sunset each day until month is completed. Young children, persons who are ill or traveling, and women who are menstruating, pregnant, or breastfeeding exempted from fasting. Pork and alcoholic beverages strictly prohibited. Only fish with fins and scales are allowed. Meat products allowed if *halal* (a special method to kill an animal) used.

Sikhs: No dietary restrictions; however, some may fast or refrain from eating meat products. Smoking and alcohol consumption generally discouraged.

* **Food prescriptions.** Those who believe in Ayurvedic medicine (mainly Hindus, Sikhs and some Muslims) classify food as "hot" or "cold." Concept of hot and cold not related to actual temperature but to food content. Hot foods prescribed in winter climate for such "cold" diseases as arthritis, respiratory tract infection, gastrointestinal problems, and circulatory problems. Fever and surgery considered a cold state. Examples of "hot" foods: all kinds of meat and fish, eggs, yogurt, honey, most oils, nuts and seeds, most herbs, and spices. "Cold" foods must be eaten during hot weather (e.g., milk, butter, cheese, most vegetables and fruits, some grains and legumes such as wheat, rice, barley, and lentils). Also believe certain foods are incompatible when eaten together such as fish and milk, meat and milk, sour fruits and milk. Believe that eating incompatible foods leads to production of toxins in body.

Fasting recommended for fever, cold, constipation, or arthritic pain. For normal healthy individual, warm water fast one day a week advised to rest digestive system.

Symptom Management

* **Pain.** *Darad* is term used to express pain in
  many South Asian languages. Would
  understand numerical scale to quantify
  pain. Hindu and Sikh patients will
  accept narcotics for pain. Muslim
  patients may refuse narcotics for mild
  to moderate pain, as narcotics forbidden in their religion; however, usually
  accepted for severe pain. Some South
  Asians may prefer taking analgesics via
  IM route. Many South Asians prefer
  home remedies to manage certain
  acute pain such as muscle pain and
  joint inflammation secondary to physical trauma. For pain secondary to surgical incision or other chronic illnesses
  such as cancer, arthritis, etc., analgesics prescribed by Western physician
  usually taken. Common home remedies include: mustard paste poultice
  applied to painful muscle and tumeric
  paste warmed and applied on piece of
  gauze to painful joint and wrapped
  with bandage overnight.

* **Dyspnea.** *Sans Ukhrna* describes breathlessness.
  May get very anxious and hyperventi-
  late as dyspnea also considered sign
  of death. Will accept oxygen with
  some explanation. Need to be
  approached in calm manner. Some
  may use home remedies such as
  licorice and ginger tea.

* **Nausea/vomiting.** *Ulti* (nausea) and vomiting
  indicates toxins in stomach which
  body must eliminate. Vomiting sometimes induced for therapeutic reasons
  in disorders such as chest congestion,
  asthma, indigestion, and edema. No
  medical treatment sought for
  nausea/vomiting initially, except
  person is encouraged to refrain from
  eating to rest gastrointestinal tract,
  and may be offered herbs and spices
  such as black pepper and/or dill seeds

* **Constipation/diarrhea.** *Kabz* (constipation);
  Julab (diarrhea). Believed that
  constipation causes abdominal disten-
  tion and discomfort, headache, and
  bad breath. To relieve constipation,
  one teaspoon of *ghee* (clarified butter)
  mixed with hot milk and taken at bedtime. Enemas generally accepted. For
  diarrhea, paste of fresh ginger mixed
  with buttermilk taken orally. Black
  coffee, cumin, or nutmeg also thought
  to cure diarrhea.

* **Fatigue**. Individuals who complain of *thakan lagna* (fatigue) advised to get enough rest and eat proper diet. Taking hot bath or shower and drinking warm glass of milk with some sugar just before bedtime believed to promote sleep and alleviate fatigue.

* **Depression.** *Dil uddas hona* in Hindi, Urdu, Punjabi, and Gujrati languages. May be considered sign of spiritual unhappiness. Some may resort to many prayers and meditation. Those who believe in Ayurvedic therapy may learn to perform Yoga exercises. In extreme or psychotic depression, help of psychiatrist or spiritual healer may be sought.

* **Self-care for symptom management.** Usually prompt in responding to symptoms causing discomfort. Tend to rely on home remedies rather than Western medications to alleviate symptoms. Medical advice sought as last resort.

Birth Rituals/Care of the New Mother/Baby

* **Pregnancy.** Pregnancy considered healthy state. Pregnant woman's mother and mother-in-law play important role in offering advice to mother. Expectant mother allowed to perform usual tasks except heavy lifting and protected from emotional stress and shock. Those who believe in Ayurvedic practice consider pregnancy a hot state and encourage foods that have cooling effect such as milk products, fruits, and vegetables. Hot foods such as meat, eggs, nuts, herbs, and spices must be avoided, especially during first trimester, as they are believed to cause miscarriage. With greater emphasis on preventive health practices and health education, prenatal care becoming common.

* **Labor practices.** Most South Asians accept delivery by trained health professional. At times, home deliveries may be preferred. Mothers encouraged to walk during labor to help dilatation of cervix and descent of fetus. Light meals advised during labor. Pain medications usually not encouraged as may delay time of delivery. Fathers usually not present at delivery but remain within reach in case of an emergency. After birth of baby, sex of child not told to mother until after placenta delivered. In some families, male

children greatly favored and birth of girl may cause mother to become emotionally upset, which may inhibit uterine contractions and obstruct delivery of placenta

* **Role of the laboring woman during birth process.** Laboring woman usually assumes passive role and follows instructions from health care providers or family members. If primipara, may be frightened and anxious. Moaning, grunting, and screaming acceptable.

* **Role of the father and other family members during birth process.** Female family member stays with mother during labor for emotional support. Father usually waits outside labor room; at times, may be anxious about condition of mother and baby. After baby is born, shown first to mother and then to father and other accompanying family members. In Muslim families, father or grandfather recites *Azan* in right ear and *Iqama* in left ear of newborn baby. This is done to confirm that the child is Muslim.

* **Vaginal vs. cesarean section.** Vaginal delivery usually preferred; however, would accept cesarean section if necessary.

* **Breastfeeding.** Breastfeeding encouraged from six months to two or three years. Working mothers may combine breastfeeding with formula for convenience. Breastfeeding mothers encouraged to eat nutritious meals for sufficient good quality milk.

* **Birth recuperation.** New mother and baby are expected to remain at home for 40 days. During this period, mother expected to get adequate rest and is offered special foods along with regular meals (e.g., *katlu* [(by Gujrati-speaking women) and *panjiri* (by Punjabi-speaking women]). This dish prepared by frying whole wheat flour in butter and adding sugar, almonds, pistachios, and a powder made of different herbs (purchased from Indian grocery store). Most of ingredients in *katlu* or *panjiri* have hot effects and are believed to restore energy that mother lost during birth process. Back massages with warm oil also common. Strongly emphasized that mother keep herself warm. May take a bath only once a week but can take partial baths and

wash perineal area with warm water every time she eliminates.

During 40 days of recuperation, relatives and friends visit to congratulate family and bring gifts for newborn. Party may be held to celebrate birth. Muslim family may perform ceremony of *Aqiqah* at party, where newborn's head is shaved, one or two goats sacrificed, and alms distributed to poor.

* **Problems with baby.** If problem with baby, mother should be told first. If serious illness, father or mother-in-law may be approached first. However, doctor is expected to reveal diagnosis; nurse's opinion generally accepted for management of ongoing problem.

* **Male and female circumcision.** Muslims: male circumcision a religious ritual that must be done before age of seven years.

    Hindus and Sikhs: male circumcision may be performed for health reasons.

    Female circumcision never practiced in any South Asian religious group.

Death Rituals

* **Preparation.** Concept of death well accepted among South Asians. Hindus, Muslims, and Sikhs believe that body dies, but soul remains alive and is immortal. Hindus and Sikhs also believe in reincarnation. Unusual to inform dying person of impending death. Family members told first about imminent death; up to them to decide whether to tell dying person. Discuss death openly with family, and offer advice to surviving younger members.

* **Home vs. hospital.** Strongly favored that death occur at home in presence of all family members. Family may wish to perform some religious rituals at time of death.

* **Special needs.** If death is imminent, family members and relatives must be called and be allowed to stay at bedside. Muslim families may offer special prayers for dying person to ease suffering. Some families may wish to call spiritual leader who prays for dying person and gives holy water to drink to purify body internally just before death. Surviving family members express their grief openly by mourning

and crying. Hindu family of deceased mourns for 40 days; Muslims mourn for three days, but hold periodic memorial gatherings (e.g., one week later, one month later, etc.).

* **Care of the body.** Muslims: As person dies, the body, arms, and legs are straightened, eyes closed, toes fastened together with bandage, and body covered with a sheet. The body then washed ritually just before burial. Body buried as soon as possible after death.

  Hindus and Sikhs: the body is washed by close family members, dressed in new clothes, and prepared for cremation. Hindus save ashes of cremated body until they can be thrown in Ganges (sacred river in India).

* **Attitudes toward organ donation.** Hindus, Muslims, and Sikhs do not allow organ donation.

* **Attitudes toward autopsy.** Most South Asians would not agree to autopsy unless absolutely necessary. Muslims would request that, if autopsy is performed, organs must be returned to body afterward.

Family Relationships

* **Composition/structure.** Extended family system common but in North America, some South Asians prefer to live in nuclear families. Extended family composed of grandparents, their sons and families, and unmarried daughters. Daughter usually expected to move in with husband's family after marriage. Same gender marriages not allowed.

* **Decision making.** Male family member, usually eldest son, has decision-making power in family. However, decisions rarely made in isolation; other family members consulted and their opinion considered before any final decision is made.

* **Spokesperson.** Father, eldest son, or any other male person in family.

* **Gender issues.** Sex roles are well defined. Men primarily responsible for all activities outside home and female for all activities within boundaries of home.

* **Caring role.** Mother, wife, daughter, or any other female relative usually assume caretaking role.

* **Expectations of and for children.** Children expected to obey their parents. Taught

to behave well and respect others, especially elders, work hard, and be religious. Treated affectionately and pampered but only to a certain extent. Quite acceptable to punish children for misbehavior. Children rarely make decisions independently. Opinion of an elder or an authority figure sought and usually carries much weight in any decision making. Children often rely on parents' decision for career choice. In homeland, greater emphasis given to vocational training than formal education. Children often encouraged to take their father's/grandfather's occupations.

* **Expectation of and for elders.** Elders very much respected in South Asian families. Younger family members not supposed to boast around or belittle elderly. Mere presence of elder family member considered blessing from God. Children and grandchildren advised to be grateful to elderly as they are believed to be reason for one's physical existence. Demands of elderly parents or grandparents are fulfilled even if it means sacrificing own wishes. Elders usually live with their children (preferably married sons) and grandchildren. Sometimes babysit and also teach cultural values and religion to their grandchildren.

* **Expectations of adults in caring for children and elders.** Adult female family members responsible for care of sick children and elders. Sick individuals admitted to hospital only if seriously ill or requiring medical interventions for complex illnesses. If sick child or elderly parent has chronic health problem and requires constant attendance of caregiver, female family member expected to care for individual at home.

* **Expectations of visitors.** In hospital, usually close female family member prefers to stay with sick individual and wishes to participate in care. Other family members visit patient frequently and may like to bring food. At times, relatives may visit patient unannounced, which may disturb the patient's comfort. Nurse may take an advocacy role in telling relatives to be considerate of patient's rest.

Spiritual/Religious Orientation

* **Primary religious/spiritual affiliation.** Most
   South Asians follow Hinduism, Islam,
   or Sikhism. Some follow practice of
   Zoroastrianism, Judaism, Jainism,
   Buddhism, or Christianity.

* **Usual religious/spiritual practices.** Hindus:
   worship many gods and goddesses.
   Believe in caste system, in which society is divided into hierarchy of four
   social classes: *Brahmins* (priest class),
   Kshatriyas (warrior class), *Vaishyas*
   (merchant class), and *Sudras* (laborer
   class). Untouchable class has been
   legally abolished but still influences
   social relations. An individual inherits
   a class at birth from parents. Birth in a
   particular caste believed to be predetermined, based on one's *Karma* in previous lives. It is one's religious duty
   (*dharma*) to adopt occupation and
   behavior that fit one's social class.
   Hindus worship in temple (*Mandir*) or
   at home. Part of their religious practice
   consists of reading from holy scripture,
   Vedas.

   Muslims: Believe in one God.
   Religious practices include: Prayers
   after ritual ablution five times daily at
   home or in congregation at mosque;
   fasting during month of *Ramazan*; giving alms (*Zakaat*); and reciting verses
   from holy book, the Koran.

   Sikhs: Believe in one God and
   equality of all people. *Guru Granth* is
   holy scripture of Sikhs. They sing
   hymns from *Guru Granth* in congregation at Sikh temple and offer
   prayers daily.

* **Use of spiritual healing/healers.** In homeland, South Asians may prefer a *Hakim*
   (homeopathic physician) or an
   Ayurvedic doctor. In Western countries, physicians generally well accepted and contacted for curing illness.
   However, many South Asians also
   believe in spiritual healing. For example, Hindus believe that recitation of
   charms and performance of certain ritual acts will eliminate diseases, ene-
   mies, sins, and demons. Many believe
   that Yoga eliminates certain physical
   and mental illnesses. Muslims believe
   that recitation of certain verses from
   Koran eliminates illnesses or eases suffering. Muslims sometimes visit shrine
   of spiritually elevated person and give

Author

Rozina Rajwani, RN, MSN currently teaches at the University of British Columbia, School of Nursing. She is first generation Indo-Canadian who immigrated to Canada in 1990 from Pakistan. She wishes to acknowledge contributions of Dr. Joan Anderson, Ms. Naz Karmali, Ms. Yasmin Kassam, and Ms. Nabdeep Sangra.

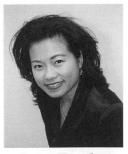

Susan Farrales

Cultural/Ethnic Identity

*   **Preferred term.** Vietnamese people. Time of arrival in U.S. determines foundation of knowledge in U.S Vietnamese. Derogatory to address them as "boat people," "refugees," or "fresh off boat" (F.O.B.).

*   **History of immigration.**

    1975–77   Variety of different types of Vietnamese people who fled via South China Sea: people with higher education and certain professional skills, families from wealthy background or with relations to American government, and generally intact families. This group acculturated more easily in U.S. and became financially self-sufficient.

    1980–1986 Known as "boat people" or "refugees." Escaped on their own to seek freedom. Some were enlisted men in South Vietnamese armed forces, fishermen, or traders. May have spent time in refugee camps. Included subpopulation of Vietnamese ethnic Chinese.

*   **Map page.** *See Appendix C, p. 1.*

Communication

*   **Major language and dialects.** Three major languages: Vietnamese (*Bac, Nam, Hue* dialects), French, and Chinese. However, they may be able to speak only French and/or Chinese. Vietnam's traditional major cities are Hanoi, Hue, and Saigon (Ho Chi Minh City). People from Hanoi speak with *Bac* accent. This is very common and known as proper way to speak Vietnamese. People from Saigon speak with *Nam* accent. People from other

parts of country may be proficient in French. Because of American involvement between 1960-1970, some people adopted English as second language. Chinese influence also spread overtly among people of Vietnam.

* **Literacy assessment.** Most Vietnamese people from first group of immigrants can understand simple English; Chinese or French may be used. Second group of immigrants and elderly will need help in translation. If patient unable to understand or read English, usually someone from family will assist with translation.

* **Nonverbal communication.** Gentle touch may be appropriate when having conversation. However, touch in communication more limited among older more traditional people, but approaches American norm among youths. Head may be considered sacred and feet profane; be careful in what order touched. Respect shown by avoiding eye contact with those of "higher status" (i.e., age, education, gender)—nurses and doctors highly respected. Respect portrayed by slightly bowing head, by using both hands in giving something to another. Personal space more distant than in Euro-Americans.

* **Use of interpreters.** Interpreter important, especially to elders and second group of immigrants. Family member may be used as interpreter, but one must remember sensitivity of subject to be discussed with patient or close member of family and be careful about gender (e.g., gynecologic care).

* **Greetings.** In formal setting, family name (last name) mentioned first; however, in casual conversation, prefer to be called by given name (first name) plus title (Mrs. plus first name). Elderly people shown respect by gentle bow. Caregiver should not shake woman's hand unless she offers her hand first. Vietnamese greet with smile and bow.

* **Tone of voice.** Typically soft spoken. Raising tone of voice and pointing finger sign of disrespect. Vietnamese use indirectness and restraint rather than confrontation in expressing interpersonal disagreement, and open expression of emotions may be considered bad taste

* **Orientation toward time.** Frequently fashionable to be late to social functions, b

understand importance of keeping
appointments. Include telephone number to call if need to cancel or be late.
Emphasize importance of appointments
and medication schedule. Usually
compliant with expectations of
health providers.

* **Consents.** Explain procedures and tests as
precisely and simply as possible. May
nod head affirmatively to acknowledge
that they heard; yet may not understand or approve. If possible, ask
patient to verbalize what was
explained to verify understanding.
Might hesitate to ask questions in
group setting; therefore, allow patient
to ask questions individually.

* **Privacy.** May open up to nurses and doctors
on one-to-one basis. If patient
requests family presence, important
to include them.

* **Serious or terminal illness.** Do not tell patient
without consulting head of family.
Often family will not want patient to
be stressed or worry even more.

Activities of Daily Living

* **Modesty.** Very modest, especially women.
Provide private room for examination.
Offer hospital gowns, robes, and pants
to everyone.

* **Skin care.** Prefer to shower daily in morning,
if no surgical sites prohibit. Good
personal hygiene very important,
especially peri-care; some prefer
soap and water after urination,
especially women.

* **Hair care.** Wash daily except after birth.
Under no circumstances should hair be
wet at night (can cause headaches).

* **Nail care.** Kept clean.

* **Toileting.** Will insist on using bathroom rather
than bedpan or urinal for privacy;
women do peri-wash, especially
before bedtime.

* **Special clothing/amulets.** If Catholic, use
religious rosary beads or figure of saint.
If Buddhist, incense usually lit.

* **Self-care.** Personal hygiene important to
patient; prefer to do it themselves. If
unable, prefer family member of same
sex to assist with care. Remember that
privacy and modesty are major issues
when in hospital. Ambulation and pulmonary toilet may be problem; therefore, need to reinforce and emphasize.

* **Role of the laboring woman during birth process.** Expectant mothers "suffer in silence"; therefore, offer lots of reassurance and comfort measures. Personal hygiene important (i.e., changing vaginal pads and keeping peri-anal area clean and dry). Most women moan or grunt when suffering. Screaming unusual. Lots of support expected from patient's mother, sister, or another close female relative.

* **Role of the father and other family members during birth process.** Fathers who attended childbirth classes may want to stay in labor room. Father expected to remain accessible; however, assumes passive role during birth process. Female family member preferred as labor coach.

* **Vaginal vs. cesarean section.** Vaginal delivery highly preferred.

* **Breastfeeding.** Traditional method of infant feeding is breastfeeding for one year. During lactation, mother adheres to restricted diet, avoiding "cold" or "windy" foods. For first 12 to 18 months, infant's diet introduced with thin gruels followed by thicker porridges made from neutral foods. Bottle feeding may be used.

* **Birth recuperation.** Care of postpartum woman seen as crucial. New mother expected to be with baby at all times. New mother freed from household work and provided with lots of rest and nourishing soup. Not allowed to take full shower for 2 to 4 weeks. However, sponge bath acceptable. Peri-care very important. Female family member will be around house to help new mother. Many women return to their mother's home to recuperate.

* **Problems with the baby.** Best to consult father or other family support person; that person will then decide who will tell new mother. Best to have doctor present when news brought to new mother.

* **Male and female circumcision.** Female circumcision never performed. Male circumcision varies, based on beliefs, economic status, and other circumstances.

Death Rituals

* **Preparation.** Inform head of family, usually parents or eldest children, in private room. DNR (Do Not Resusitate)a

sensitive issue and decision made by entire family. Priest or monk may come to provide assistance.

* **Home vs. hospital.** For acute illness, will prefer that patient stay in hospital. However, if patient suffers from terminal illness, prefer to die at home with dignity.

* **Special needs.** For Catholic families, religious medallion, rosary beads, or other spiritual objects such as figure of saint kept close to patient. Family may start praying. Priest present in room. For Buddhist families, incense lit in room and monk present to start religious ritual. Important to allow family extra time with deceased patient. May start crying loudly and uncontrollably.

* **Care of the body.** The body highly respected. Certain families may want to wash the body themselves; others might want it left as is. Spiritual/religious rite usually takes place in room.

* **Attitudes toward organ donation.** The body given high respect; organ donation not allowed. Cremation preferred by Buddhists. Immigrants of longer duration or those more acculturated may accept organ donations.

* **Attitudes toward autopsy.** Same as above. If necessary under certain circumstances, entire family will decide.

Family Relationships

* **Composition/structure.** Highly family-oriented; may be extended or nuclear family. Sometimes two or three generations in one household. May not be tolerant or supportive of gay/lesbian sibling; first immigrants more supportive than second group. Acculturation caused shift from extended to nuclear family system and decision making may be confined to spousal couple because they no longer have duty to seek advice and consent from parental families.

* **Decision making/spokesperson.** Father or eldest son is family spokesperson. Wives who are not wage earners demonstrate more subordinate patterns of decision making. Women tend to continue attitude that husbands have legitimate right to make final decisions; usually will withdraw from spousal conflict to maintain harmony within family.

* **Gender issues.** Men decision makers and support for family. Their job to carry out heavy-duty chores and to be strong in crisis.

    Women prepare all meals, whether employed or not. Do most of household chores unless children old enough to help. When women get jobs more easily than men, however, traditional roles and family relationships strained.

* **Caring role.** Women in family responsible for ill patient. Women act as primary care providers at bedside, regardless of patient's sex. Expected to pamper patient with daily bath and meals.

* **Expectations of and for children**. When children young, parents look after them, and when parents get old, children look after them. Children well sheltered by parents. Expected to obey and honor parents and respect elders; taught to be honest, quiet, and polite.

    Strong emphasis on education. Parents push children to highest level in education, especially when they didn't have opportunity themselves. Some intergenerational conflicts with children acculturating to American norms or when child must serve as spokesperson/interpreter.

* **Expectations of and for elders.** Stay with family for support and comfort. Elders highly respected by all age groups.

    Depending on socioeconomic status and lifestyle, elders expected to prepare meals and take care of grandchildren while wife and husband work.

* **Expectations of adults in caring for children and elders.** Adults expected to assume full responsibility for sick member at home. Traditionally, sick elders cared for at home, unless circumstances make it necessary to place them in nursing home. Being institutionalized believed to be disrespectful to elderly.

* **Expectation of visitors.** As mentioned above, female family member expected to stay at bedside for comfort and support. Private room recommended. Because Vietnamese are family-centered, many family members and friends come to visit.

Spiritual/Religious Orientation
* **Primary religious/spiritual affiliation.**
    Two predominant religions are Catholicism and Buddhism; heaviest

concentrations of Roman Catholics from northern part of Vietnam. Also many Protestants. Other religions a blend of Theravada Buddhism, local and ancestor spirit worship, Confucionism and Taoism.

* **Usual religious/spiritual practices.** Catholics recite rosary or read prayers/novena. Call for chaplain daily. Buddhists practice act of *Dana* (or generosity), believed to return to them in future as *karma*. Theravada Buddhism holds that individuals must seek their own salvation. Believe in reincarnation and in an ultimate Nirvana. Pray silently among themselves.

* **Use of spiritual healing/healers.** When one becomes ill, priest or monk visits patient, and/or family, necessitating privacy.

Illness Beliefs

* **Causes of physical illness.** Four types of explanations for illness. "Natural" cause attributes illness to natural or immediately visible circumstances such as rotten food. Chinese-Vietnamese explanations for illness based on traditional Chinese philosophy of balance between *ying* and *yang*, hot and cold. Supernatural explanations for illness include punishment for personality fault or violation of religious taboo. Western biomedical causes, such as "germs," also explain illness.

* **Causes of mental illness.** Mental illness caused by disruption of harmony in individual. Some believe mental illness caused by ancestral spirit coming back to haunt them because of past bad behavior.

* **Causes of genetic defects.** Accept loved ones unconditionally, but believe genetic defect in family is God's punishment for wrong behavior. Will care for child at home and be very protective due to shame.

* **Sick role.** Patient assumes passive role; cared for by family member. Patient well taken care of, which includes having everything own way.

* **Home and folk remedies.** Treated with herbal medicine, spiritual practices, and acupuncture. Other conventional Vietnamese health practices include cupping, coin rubbing, or pinching skin. Western health providers have

mistaken coin rubbing for evidence of child abuse because resembles large blue-red mark on skin, similar to a bruise, but with a long, wide mark. This done to create area for offending wind to escape. Cupping involves applying a glass from which oxygen has been removed to afflicted skin area. Suction created by lack of oxygen in glass causes skin to rise up and turn bluish. Other practices include inhaling aromatic oils (e.g., eucalyptus), herbal teas, or wearing strings tied on body.

* **Acceptance of procedures.** If blood needed, family member willing to donate. Must explain slowly and clearly. Some might want to consult another physician for second opinion.

* **Care seeking.** Believe in both Western biomedicine and folk medicine. Some believe traditional healers can exorcise evil spirits. With certain conditions, treatment must fit illness (e.g., spiritual cure for spiritual illness).

Health Practices

* **Concept of health.** Based on principles of harmony and balance within themselves.

  Being overweight not of great concern—instead, positive sign of good socioeconomic status and contentment.

* **Health promotion and prevention.** To promote health is to understand holistic concept that encompasses physical, spiritual, emotional, and social factors. Consuming lots of fresh vegetables, fruits, fish, and meat promote good health. Keeping oneself clean looking also promotes good health. Maintaining warm environment prevents suffering from muscle or bone aches. Exercise not regular part of daily activities.

* **Screening.** Have respect for medical authority and will only seek screening if emphasized by doctor or nurse. Be sure to get family member involved in emergency screening.

Selected References

Fox, P. (1991). Stress related to family change among Vietnamese refugees. *Journal of Community Health Nursing*, 8(1), 45-56.

Gold, S. (1992). Mental health and illness in Vietnamese refugees. *Western Journal of Medicine, 157,* 290-294.

Shanahan, M., & Brayshaw, D. L. (1995). Are nurses aware of the differing health care needs of Vietnamese patients? *Journal of Advanced Nursing, 22*(3), 456-464.

Stauffer, R. (1995). Vietnamese Americans. In J. Geiger & R. Davidhizar (Eds.), *Transcultural nursing: Assessment and intervention* (pp. 441-472). St. Louis: Mosby.

Author

Susan Farrales, RN, BSN is a Clinical Nurse II of Pediatrics in the Medical Center at the University of California, San Francisco. Born in Vietnam, her mother is Vietnamese and her father Filipino. They immigrated to the U.S. in 1975.

Trinidadians, Jamaicans, & Barbadians

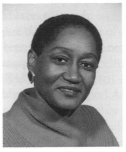

Patricia St. Hill

Cultural/Ethnic Identity

* **Preferred terms.** West Indian, or more ideally Jamaican, Trinidadian, Barbadian, etc., depending on particular Caribbean Island from which individual has migrated. However, this cultural group, often referred to as an "ethnic melting pot," is highly ethnically diverse, with individuals of East Indian, Chinese, Caucasian, and Black/African ancestry, many of whom have chosen to retain their ancestral heritage. These secondary ethnic or cultural identities may also emerge or be claimed by certain individuals within this population.

  Dominicans, another group from Caribbean region, share many cultural beliefs and practices with Trinidadians, Jamaicans, and Barbadians. However, Dominicans, with long history of Spanish rule, speak Spanish and have Latin flavor to their culture whereas other groups who were former British colonies do not.

* **History of immigration.**

1820	First written documentation of West Indian migration to U.S. That year, 164 individuals reportedly migrated to U.S., which had boundless need for manpower to build railroads as well as many other labor needs.
1901–1920	Increased West Indian migration to U.S., coinciding with industrialization and urbanization of American society and its ever increasing needs for manpower to fuel booming industrial economy.
1941–1950	Migration upsurge in response to America's increasing need for temporary agricultural workers and enactment of Mexican Bracero Program, permitting easy

and fears surrounding notion of death
and dying in this culture.

Activities of Daily Living

*   **Modesty.** Extreme modesty about "private"
    body parts. Much embarrassment asso-
    ciated with idea of having to expose
    one's body to a stranger (practitioner).
    This embarrassment or "shame," as
    West Indians say, heightened if health
    provider of opposite gender, and made
    even worse if both younger and of
    opposite gender. Extra measures
    should be taken to minimize patient's
    body exposure and create safe,
    trusting environment.

*   **Skin care.** Observes good personal hygiene.
    Showers daily and may shower again at
    night or perform good peri-care, an
    activity referred to as "washing off." If
    ill, particularly if spiking fever or suf-
    fering from very bad cold, will refrain
    from taking showers, fearing that body
    will be exposed to "chill" or "draft."

*   **Hair care.** Hair washing by Black West Indian
    female done about once a week, in
    effort to preserve natural oils in her
    naturally dry hair type. Individuals
    with Chinese, East Indian or Spanish
    ancestry, having different hair texture,
    will wash hair more frequently.

*   **Nail care.** Preferred nail lengths vary.
    Maintaining clean nails important,
    however.

*   **Toileting.** Observes good hygiene. Very strict
    about hand washing, especially after
    using bathroom facilities and before
    preparing or touching foods. Will not
    object to using urinal and/or bedpan, i
    indicated, but requires privacy.

*   **Special clothing/amulets.** May wear cross on
    chain around neck, or have pin of
    saint attached to clothing. Leave such
    items in place if not interfering with
    treatment since they give patient extr
    sense of protection.

*   **Self-care.** Family member, usually mother or
    grandmother, will stay at bedside and
    assist or provide personal care when
    patient is unable to provide own care.
    If staff provides care, same gender
    provider preferable.

Food Practices

*   **Usual meal pattern.** Three major meals per
    day customary, but will snack betweer

meals. In West Indies, lunch largest meal of day, equivalent to dinner in U.S. society. Dinner much lighter meal, comparable to breakfast. Typical dinner consists of bread or homemade biscuits (bakes) and hot beverage (tea or chocolate).

Since West Indian cooking typically very spicy, patient may keep bottle of hot sauce and/or other Caribbean spices at bedside to add to hospital meals. RN should advise patient and visitors about any dietary restrictions for patient.

* **Food beliefs and rituals.** Hot foods served hot and cold foods cold. Have primarily hot soups and broths when ill and avoid use of ice.

* **Usual diet.** Rice a staple in West Indian diet. Rice with various stewed meats and gravies comprise typical lunch. On Sundays, lunch a special, much larger meal consisting of more expensive foods not normally served during week. Minimal concerns in this culture about limiting fatty foods, red meat intake, and cholesterol levels. Cooking with coconut oil, extremely high in cholesterol, very common for enhancing flavor of foods.

* **Fluids.** Consistent with warm, dry climate in West Indies, West Indians drink significant amount of water and homemade fruit juices, served with ice. Drink only warm liquids when ill, however.

* **Food prohibitions.** Eating acid fruits or drinking acid fruit juices immediately after coming out of sun, while body is warm, thought to be bad—capable of "turning the blood acid."

For religious reasons, most West Indians will not eat meat on Fridays during Lent, especially on Good Friday. Fish traditionally served on these days. For people of East Indian heritage following Moslem and Hindu religions, pork or beef prohibited.

* **Food prescriptions.** Liver prescribed for combatting anemia or to "build up the blood." To regain strength or "build up the body" following an illness, large amounts of soups and broths made from various animal organs and parts prescribed. They include: cow foot soup, fish head soup, and tripe soup made from segments of cow's stomach.

Since family members can be expected to bring these foods to help patient recuperate more quickly, necessary to make family aware of patient's dietary restrictions.

Symptom Management

*   **Pain.** Pain signals onset of illness. Most people tend to try various home remedies before seeking medical attention. Typical among home remedies used are herbal or "bush teas" made from various wild bushes or parts of plants or trees, including bark, leaves, flowers, and roots. In addition to teas, various ointments and balms may also be applied to site of pain.

    For many West Indians, prescription medications feared to cause possible harm or addiction. Hence, when forced to take prescription medications, tend to discontinue use of drugs as soon as symptoms disappear. RN should emphasize importance of completing full course of medication.

    Given a choice of medications, oral medications more likely to be chosen over IM, IV or rectal modes; likelihood of greater compliance with oral meds.

*   **Dyspnea.** Viewed as serious medical condition generally associated with asthma, for which conventional medical help will be sought. Will accept use of oxygen and opioids to control dyspnea and, if asked, will express discomfort experienced in breathing, using words to describe discomfort level.

*   **Nausea/vomiting.** Generally associated with having eaten something that "disagreed with you." Customary to drink hot tea and avoid eating solid foods as long as episode of nausea and vomiting lasts.

*   **Constipation/diarrhea.** Change in bowel function generally attributed to certain food or foods one has eaten. In fact, certain foods are thought to cause constipation. Insufficient fluid intake or lack of exercise not recognized as causing constipation. If in discomfort patient will report constipation to RN although not a topic generally discussed. Will accept whatever medication is prescribed. However, may be reluctant to have enema, but will comply if importance explained.

296

At home, constipation relief calls for "purge" or "wash out," using harsh laxatives such as epsom salts or castor oil. Typically, few teaspoons of epsom salts dissolved in small amount of water and drunk, or few teaspoons of castor oil would be taken for same purpose.

* **Fatigue.** Sign that person is "run down" or anemic and needs nourishing foods to "build him up." Will report symptoms of fatigue in very expressive terms and be willing to accept medications to improve condition, preferably tonics.

* **Depression.** May hesitate to report to RN. As with all mental illness, depression stigmatized and seen as sign of personal weakness. If asked, however, likely to admit "feeling under the weather" and describe signs and symptoms, but not very likely to use actual word "depression."

* **Self-care for symptom management.** Will respond to symptoms by seeking out appropriate herbal tea, based on symptoms experienced. Also, will take to bed or simply decrease household duties until condition improves.

Birth Rituals/Care of the New Mother/Baby

* **Pregnancy care.** Prenatal care increasingly becoming norm for women in larger Caribbean Islands. Prenatally, woman pays close attention to diet, avoiding foods thought to be bad for baby, while making sure to include those that will nourish and fatten baby. Closely monitoring weight gain during pregnancy generally not an important consideration. More weight gained by pregnant woman, healthier both mother and baby thought to be.

* **Labor practices.** Due to limited number of licensed MDs, midwives' attendance at births still quite common. During labor, woman encouraged to keep walking. Many known to proceed with housework during early stages of labor. As contractions become closer and labor pains intensify, midwife will be called and begin monitoring and coaching woman through delivery. Not customary for husband or male partner to witness or participate in delivery. Close female friend or relative will be present to support woman during labor.

* **Role of the laboring woman during birth process.** Woman's role during birth process somewhat passive, following instructions given. To maintain dignity, she "suffers in silence" during labor. Stoically endures labor pains, too ashamed to cry out loud as contractions get closer and labor pains more severe.
* **Role of the father and other family members during birth process.** Traditionally, father not present or involved; may go out with friends, eagerly awaiting news of birth, or may remain at home to care for small children in family.
* **Vaginal vs. cesarean section.** Vaginal delivery much preferred over cesarean section and also much more common.
* **Breastfeeding.** Breastfeeding customary until child about 9 months of age. For many West Indian women, this prolonged period of breastfeeding has been used as form of birth control. Today, with increasing numbers of working mothers, a combination of breast- and bottle feeding common.
* **Birth recuperation.** New mother stays in bed for approximately a week. During this time, expected to do no heavy lifting or strenuous work. Often female relative, generally woman's mother, will stay with her to assist with housework and care for infant.
* **Problems with baby.** Best to inform father of child or grandparents prior to telling mother. This allows them time to prepare mother for bad news and to be there to support her.
* **Male and female circumcision.** Male circumcision not customary in this culture. However, most parents, if asked to have male child circumcised prior to discharge, will agree. Female circumcision never practiced.

Death Rituals
* **Preparation.** Surviving partner should be informed of death as soon as possible, preferably in presence of adult children/relatives.

Often family members ask to view body of deceased in hospital bed, just as he/she died. RN may offer to call chaplain to meet with family. Most families, however, will choose to be left alone with departed loved one.

* **Home vs. hospital.** Most families will care for chronically ill/dying relative at home. Done out of sense of family obligation and loyalty as well as respect for dying relative.
* **Special needs.** When death is imminent, close friends and family will want to gather at bedside of dying person to pray and to witness loved one's passing. Staff, once making sure that patient is comfortable, should leave family to themselves.
* **Care of the body.** Not customary for family to care for or prepare body for mortuary. Hospital personnel may take over at this point.
* **Attitudes toward organ donation.** Family members not likely to agree to organ donation. Maintaining integrity of body an important consideration in this culture, given many myths surrounding death and presumed after-life.

    If organ donation request is to be made, however, health care professional should approach family discreetly and make extra effort not to put any pressure on them.
* **Attitudes toward autopsy.** Will forego autopsy if not medically necessary. Maintaining integrity of body remains important consideration.

Family Relationships

* **Composition/structure.** Nuclear family unit, often including widowed elderly parent, is customary. However, very close family ties maintained with members of extended family, and activities of individual family members will bring shame to entire family. This includes homosexuality, not accepted in this culture, and viewed as shameful and kept secret from people on outside, when possible. Often gay person, fearing family reprisal, will attempt to conceal his/her homosexuality and not readily "come out" to family.
* **Decision making.** Male traditionally head of household and thus source of power and decision making. Increasingly, however, female (especially those employed outside home) shares power and participates in decision-making process.

stress generally perceived as source of
mental illness. Less frequently, though,
that evil spirits placed on person by an
enemy responsible for mental illness.

* **Causes of genetic defects.** Genetic defects
in child frequently perceived and
explained as work of God or God's will
for that family. Such defects also some
times explained as affliction or punish
ment from God for parental sins.

* **Sick role.** Sick person expected to stay in bed
and be cared for by relatives. Also
expected to be fed nutritious foods to
rebuild resistance and body.

* **Home and folk remedies.** Use of home reme
dies remains significant and integral
part of health care in West Indies.
Herbal teas, known locally as "bush
tea," used to prevent, control, and
cure almost all ailments. For each ail
ment, there is known plant, bush,
leaf, flower, root, or bark assigned.
Strong reliance on home remedies
largely responsible for advanced stage
in which patients generally enter
health care system. If asked about
use of home remedies, patients gener
ally will disclose information to
health professional.

* **Acceptance of procedures.** In accordance
with respect for authority, most West
Indian patients generally accept
surgeries, blood transfusions,
organ transplants, and whatever
procedures suggested, if deemed
medically necessary.

* **Care seeking.** Generally seek medical atten
tion only when physically ill and
unable to perform daily tasks, or at
advanced stage of disease process.

Health Practices

* **Concept of health.** Good health defined as
absence of physical pain, ability to per
form one's usual activities, and weight
gain, even if person is overweight. In
West Indies, unlike U.S., being thin
negative phenomenon often associat
with disease. Very thin person suspect
ed of having TB or some other conta
gious disease and hence shunned.

* **Health promotion and prevention.**
Promotion and maintenance of good
health associated with eating well:
large servings of heavy foods, rich in
carbohydrates, on a scheduled basis.

Regular exercise, lowering cholesterol levels through decreased fat consumption, and lowering sugar and salt content in foods typically not among health promotion measures espoused in this society.

* **Screening.** Preventive care such as annual physicals, pap smears, and mammograms, is not customary practice for most people. West Indians very private people, easily embarrassed, who believe in keeping private matters strictly within family. Will not readily disclose information on matters of private nature such as sexual activity, history of sexually transmitted diseases or any other contagious diseases, abortions, use of alternative medical treatments, or faith healing. In screening, be sure to discreetly ask questions about these matters, which will not be readily volunteered, but which may have direct bearing on diagnosis and treatment.

Selected References

The Diagram Group. (1985). *The atlas of Central America and the Caribbean.* New York: Macmillan.

Handwerker, W. P. (1992). West Indian gender relations, family planning programs, and fertility decline. *Social Science and Medicine, 35*(10), 1245-1257.

Author

Patricia F. St. Hill, RN, MPH, PhD is currently a post-doctoral scholar at the University of Washington, Seattle. She received her PhD from the University of California, San Francisco School of Nursing where her studies and research focus were in the area of community/cross-cultural health nursing. Born on the tiny Caribbean island of Trinidad, Dr. St. Hill migrated with her family to the United States at the age of 15.

Population Tables & Maps

Nurses should familiarize themselves with the cul-
ral and sociodemographic characteristics of the most
opulous groups to whom they provide care. Locally,
ch information may be available in county or state
ealth departments, city chambers of commerce, or
iblic libraries. However, data on some groups may
ot be available.

Obtaining accurate population figures for the immi-
ant groups and their descendants in the U.S. that are
overed in this book was surprisingly difficult. The U.S.
ensus is highly inaccurate for a number of groups. The
990 Census used three major categories: **Race,**
Hispanic Origin, and **First Ancestry.** Smaller popula-
ons are grouped together in the public use Census data,
ut often inaccurately. An example is Haitians who are
lassified as "black race" rather than of West Indian
ncestry. Inaccuracies and inability to sample evenly
cross groups are due to a number of factors: some peo-
le had difficulty identifying with a Census category;
ome were afraid to participate, and others did not
nderstand why or how they should participate because
f language. Many Brazilians, for example, checked
white" because Hispanic origin (Spain/Spanish) was
naccurate and there was no specific Brazilian category.
Undocumented Brazilians avoided Census takers.
razilian population estimates by knowledgeable
gencies and the 1990 Census are widely divergent:
50,000 versus 94,023 (Margolis, 1995). Census maps
ncluded in this appendix show concentrations of
ederally recognized "minority" groups.

Another problem is that there is no easy way to
haracterize people of mixed ancestry or racial back-
round. Further, within any group, there are new immi-
rants and long-settled citizens, and it is difficult to tease
ut the very important influence of how long an individ-
al or family has been in the U.S., which strongly affects
ealth patterns. Therefore, the numbers in this table
hould not be assumed to be accurate. The table is
ntended to provide a rough idea of the relative numbers
f ethnic/racial groups described in this book.

POPULATION DATA FOR SELECTED ETHNIC GROUPS

Group	U.S. #	State #1[1]	State #2	State #3
Arab	716,391	CA: 123,933	NY: 79,600	MI: 65,906
Black/ African- American	29,930,524	NY: 2,860,590	CA: 2,198,766	TX: 2,018,543
Brazilian[2]	375,000	NY, NJ, CT: 200,000	FL: 120,000	CA: 20,000
Cambodian	149,047	CA: 71,178	MA: 13,849	WA: 10,757
Chinese	1,647,486	CA: 713,423	NY: 285,322	HI: 68,769

POPULATION DATA FOR SELECTED ETHNIC GROUPS
continued

Group	U.S. #	State #1[1]	State #2	State #3
Columbian	378,726	NY: 107,377	FL: 83,634	NJ: 52,210
Cuban	1,053,197	FL: 675,786	NJ: 87,085	NY: 77,016
Ethiopian[2]	123,000	CA	Wash., DC	NY
Filipino	1,419,711	CA: 733,941	HI: 168,232	IL: 67,383
Guatemalan	268,779	CA: 159,177	NY: 21,995	IL: 16,017
Gypsies[2]	300,000	NYC	LA, S.F. Bay Area	Cleveland, Seattle
Haitian[3]	365,000	FL: 125,000	NY: 125,000	MA: 35,000
Hmong	94,439	CA: 49,343	MN: 17,764	WI: 16,980
E. Indian	786,694	CA: 154,122	NY: 132,801	NJ: 79,367
Iranian[4]	285,000	CA	NY	Wash., DC
Japanese	866,160	CA: 320,730	HI: 252,291	NY: 36,488
Korean	797,304	CA: 259,908	NY 97,111	IL: 41,436
Mexican	13,393,208	CA: 6,070,637	TX: 3,899,518	AZ: 619,435
American Indian	1,937,391	OK: 252,132	CA: 243,736	AZ: 204,150
Nicaraguan	202,658	FL: 79,056	CA: 74,119	NY: 11,011
Pakistanis[2]	500,000	NY	Chicago, IL	CA
Puerto Rican	2,651,815	NY: 1,046,896	NJ: 304,179	FL: 240,673
Russian	2,114,506	NY: 455,162	CA: 327,675	FL: 183,244
Salvadoran	565,081	CA: 388,769	TX: 58,128	NY: 47,350
Samoan	57,679	CA: 28,320	HI: 15,000	WA: 3,589
Vietnamese	593,213	CA: 280,233	TX: 69,634	WA: 20,693
West Indian	21,058,345	NY: 452,338	FL: 226,854	NJ: 60,668

[1] This column shows the state in which the group is most po
ulous; states #2 and #3 are the second and third most populo
states.

[2] U.S. Census data for specific group either unavailable or
undercounted. Table estimates are provided by chapter auth
or others based on various sources and in-depth knowledge o
the specific population. West Indians include Haitians,
Trinidadians, Barbadians, Jamaicans.

Stepick, A., & Stepick, C. D. (1995). *Demographics of the Diaspora: Census Results of Haitians in the U.S.* Immigration and Ethnicity Institute, Florida International University.

Bozorgmehr, M. (1995). Diaspora in the postrevolutionary period. *Encyclopedia Iranica, 7,* 380-383.

Reference

Margolis, M. (1995). Brazilians and the 1990 United States Census: Immigrants, ethnicity and the undercount. *Human Organization, 54,* 52-59.

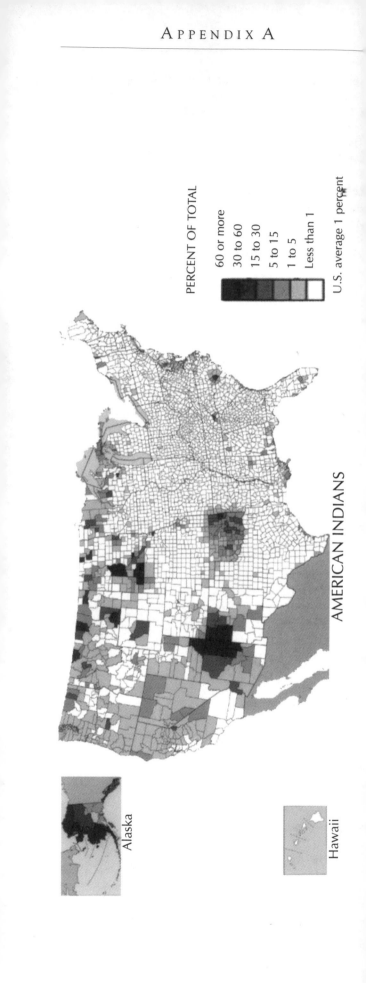

PERCENT OF TOTAL

60 or more
30 to 60
15 to 30
5 to 15
1 to 5
Less than 1

U.S. average 1 percent

AMERICAN INDIANS

Alaska

Hawaii

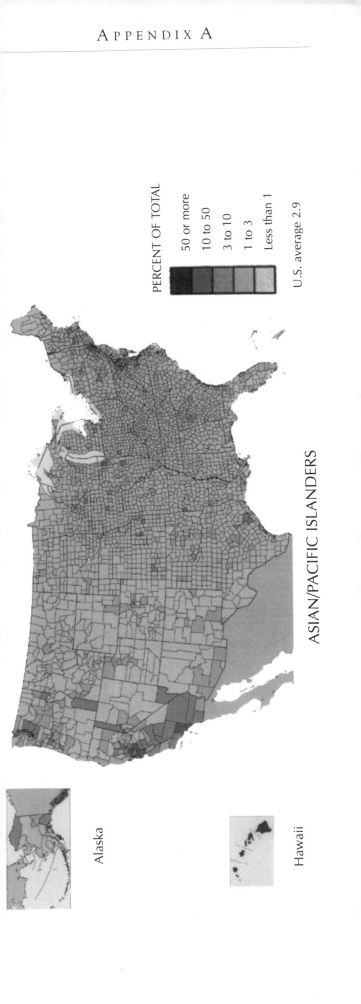

PERCENT OF TOTAL

50 or more

10 to 50

3 to 10

1 to 3

Less than 1

U.S. average 2.9

ASIAN/PACIFIC ISLANDERS

Alaska

Hawaii

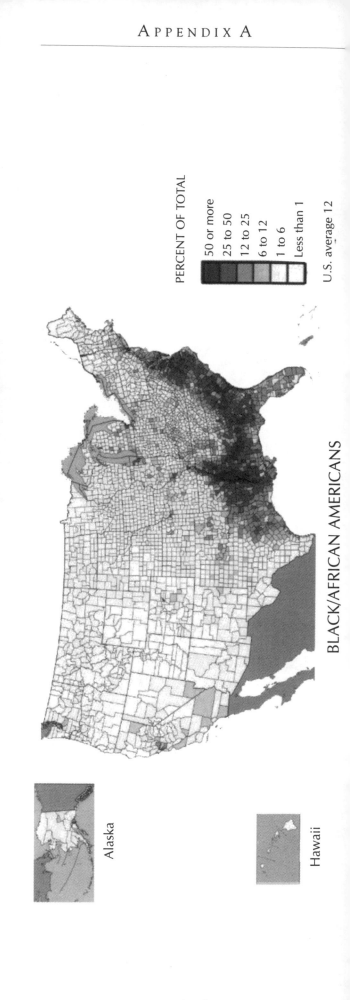

PERCENT OF TOTAL

50 or more
25 to 50
12 to 25
6 to 12
1 to 6
Less than 1

U.S. average 12

BLACK/AFRICAN AMERICANS

Alaska

Hawaii

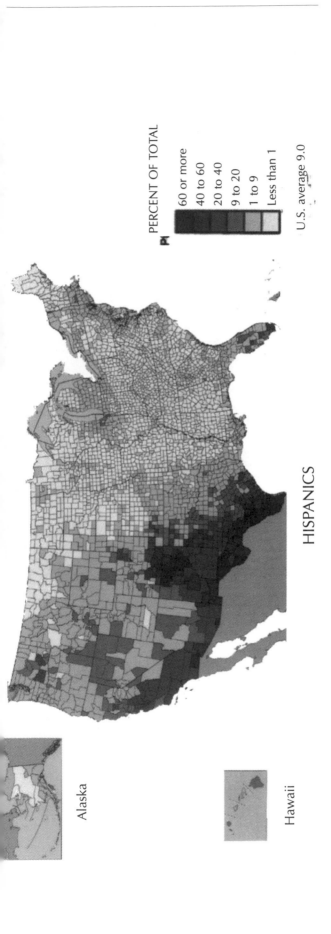

PERCENT OF TOTAL

60 or more
40 to 60
20 to 40
9 to 20
1 to 9
Less than 1

U.S. average 9.0

HISPANICS

Alaska

Hawaii

Diversity Among Spiritual and Religious Beliefs

Pamela A. Minarik,
RN, MS, FAAN

This brief overview of major religious/spiritual systems in U.S. includes beliefs, rituals and practices, and standards of conduct that influence health care. Nurses should use this chapter only as a guide to individualize care, always verifying significance of beliefs or practices for persons involved.

ADVENTIST (SEVENTH DAY)

* **Names by Which the Particular Sect is Known.** Adventist; Church of God; Seventh Day Adventist; Advent Christian Church— 783,000 members in North America.
* **Spiritual/Religious Beliefs That Explain the Presence of Health and Illness.** Bible accepted literally. Evidence of salvation is keeping of commandments. Members believe it is their duty to warn others to prepare for second coming of Christ when final rewards and punishment will be meted out. The body considered temple of God and must be kept healthy. Concerned about health and involved in health care. Healing can be accomplished both through medical intervention and divine healing. Operate one of world's largest religious health care systems, including hospitals, clinics, and medical and nursing schools. Chaplains and physicians inseparable. Emphasize physical medicine, rehabilitation, and therapeutic diets. Opposed to hypnotism.
* **Spiritual/Religious Implements.** Prayer and anointing with oil. No special sacraments or rituals at birth or death.
* **Daily Practices That Might Be Performed Frequently.** Some sects consider Saturday the Sabbath, day of worship and rest.
* **Food Requirements and Prohibitions.** Vegetarian diet encouraged. Many groups prohibit meat, shellfish, and some birds, which may result in iodine or protein deficiencies; therefore, may be important to teach about substitutes. Alcohol, coffee, and tea prohibited. Fasting practiced by some sects.

Spiritual/Religious Practices Associated with Life Transitions

* **Pregnancy and Birth.** Birth control an individual choice. Artificial insemination acceptable between husband and wife. Therapeutic abortion acceptable in cases of danger to mother, rape or incest.

Opposed to infant baptism. Adults baptized by total immersion.

* **Illness.** No restrictions on medications, blood or blood products, or vaccines. Some groups prohibit narcotics and stimulants, because the body, as temple of the Holy Spirit, should be protected. No restrictions on surgical procedures, amputations, transplants, or biopsies, although some people will refuse interventions on Friday evening and Saturday (Sabbath). Healing practices include prayer and anointing with oil. Patient may take Communion or undergo baptism.

* **Dying and Death.** Prefer prolonging life but may allow someone to die in some cases. Euthanasia not practiced. Autopsy, donation of body or organs acceptable. Disposal of body and burial are individual decisions.

* **Expected Involvement of Spiritual/Religious Practitioners in the Illness.** At request of ill person or family, pastor and elders pray and anoint ill person with oil.

* **What the Nurse Can Do to Facilitate These Specific Spiritual/Religious Practices.** Ask patient and family about their beliefs and preferences and provide suitable environment. Provide privacy and quiet for visits from pastor or elder.

AMERICAN INDIAN RELIGIONS

(contributed by LaDonna Osborne, BA)

* **Names by Which the Particular Sect is Known.** There are more than 2 million people in 300-500 different American Indian tribal groups, each with its own culture and responses to specific situations. Health care practices intertwined with religious and cultural beliefs. Common religions within traditional American Indian religions are Native American Church and Indian Baptist Church. Specific tribes follow own rituals, referred to in general terms, such as the Lakota Way or the Navajo Way. Probably as many religious beliefs as there are tribes, each with sacred songs, dance, and prayers. American Indians may belong to traditional as well as Christian church. (Also see American Indian Chapter).

* **Spiritual/Religious Beliefs That Explain the Presence of Health and Illness.** Religious ceremonies vary from tribe to tribe. Common bond among most tribes is belief in Creator. Some tribes use God and Creator interchangeably. American Indian religious traditions have been passed through the generations by

storytelling. Some tribes believe Bible a written version of "white men's stories."

Ill health results from not living in harmony or being out of balance with nature and social and supernatural environments. Religious ceremonies performed with intent of seeing, understanding, or obtaining a vision of clarity of oneself and individual issues. When Creator reveals answer to question or problem that has been pondered, then up to individual to change behavior, or take action on message received from Creator. If person does not listen or act on messages received, then individual will continue to be in pain. Sufficient physical or emotional pain will lead to necessary knowledge to begin to heal.

Some religious ceremonies rid body of impurities. A "sweat" is performed in a sweat lodge. Leader of sweat ceremony adds water to rocks, creating steam in lodge. Specific songs sung to Creator, tribute to earth, and ancestors asked to reach from heavens to earth to give wisdom, guidance, and vision. Ceremony continues for several hours with specific times set aside for singing, sharing, prayer, and silent contemplation. Spiritual as well as physical cleansing occurs as toxins are removed from body through sweat. Also a ceremony of endurance, as heat can become quite stifling. Through strong prayer and strong mind, person transcends physical discomfort and becomes receptive to wisdom of ancestors.

Within Native American Church, peyote used as sacrament. Believed that peyote gives humans visions, answers, guidance, and strength. If person is in good spiritual condition, peyote will speak to him or her. If person is "out of balance," he or she may become very ill with nausea and vomiting, viewed as cleansing. Metaphorically, person is holding onto something or not letting go, and peyote gives release.

An ill person may seek medical services through hospital or clinic as well as Medicine Man or Woman. Believed that Medicine People have capacity to heal through prayer, ceremony, and spiritual powers given by ancestors. Some diseases viewed as "non-Indian" diseases, such as diabetes, heart disease, and alcoholism, introduced by white people through diet, etc. These diseases did not traditionally exist.

* **Spiritual/Religious Implements.**
Instruments are sacred and should not be touched without permission. If ill person cannot move instruments, family member or friends may move instruments; stranger is last

resort for this task. Some common sacred instruments include:

Medicine bag: Leather pouch usually worn around neck. Contents of pouch considered sacred medicine. Medicine Bag should not be opened. Improper to ask about contents of bag.

Fan: Made of feathers, fan has handle with horsehair or white string fringe at bottom.

Staff or Prayer Staff: Staff can be of various sizes. Most commonly a length of wood. May be decorated with eagle, hawk, or owl talons, beadwork, antlers, or anything else found in nature. Staff usually held during prayer or singing of traditional religious songs.

Rattle: Rattle has handle made of gourd, turtle shells or other material. May be decorated as described above and is used during singing.

Feathers: May be single feathers or several feathers, loose, tied together or hanging from wall or ceiling, or over door. Wing of large bird may be intact.

Sections of Animals: Tribes include families or clans, e.g., wolf clan, turtle clan, or coyote clan. Members of clan may keep a skull, tail, or shell of that animal in room.

Cedar: Cedar branch or needles may be strewn about area. Used for purification.

Sage: Sage sticks usually in bundles rather than single pieces of sage and are used for purification. When burned, smells strongly like marijuana.

Cedar box: Box with handle on top, usually long and narrow. Religious instruments as well as items sacred to individual are placed in this box. Not to be opened by anyone except owner or selected individual.

Pipe: Usually a wooden shaft made with a red stone bowl. Used to smoke tobacco during prayer.

Drum: So sacred that it is unlikely to be brought into a hospital setting.

* **Daily Practices That Might Be Performed Frequently.** Prayers may be performed daily, and may include use of pipe, burning cedar, sage, or tobacco. Some tribes sprinkle ground corn on floor which can make it slippery. Prayer not usually done in public or with strangers in attendance. If hospital chaplain offers to pray aloud with family, would be unlikely for family to refuse out of respect for chaplain. However, this is an invasion of privacy unless family itself requests chaplain's attendance.

* **Food Requirements and Prohibitions.** After ceremony or prayer, common foods consumed are berries, corn, and dried meat, most likely be provided by family.

piritual/Religious Practices Associated /ith Life Transitions

* **Pregnancy and Birth.** Pregnant women continue to use religious ceremonies, sweats, and peyote during pregnancy and up until delivery.
* **Illness.** See previous section.
* **Dying and Death.** Beliefs and practices vary widely from tribe to tribe. Some tribes believe seeing an owl is omen of death. The body is sometimes prepared for burial by family members or member of tribe. After person dies, some tribes will not touch the deceased person's clothes or personal belongings. If person dies in the house, not uncommon to abandon the house forever. While death is sad experience for the living, some groups believe the deceased will join ancestors in spirit world and be happy and free of earthly bonds. Some tribes view dead person's body as simply an empty shell, while other tribes go to great lengths to prepare the body for ritual and visit the deceased.
* **Expected Involvement of Spiritual/Religious Practitioners in the Illness.** Family notifies and requests visit by their religious practitioner. Due to privacy of traditional beliefs and commitment to old ways, Medicine Man or Woman will probably not have identification defining member of the clergy. Religious practitioner may be introduced as cousin or uncle. Include elder, medicine person, or spiritual leader as colleague to assist in healing process.
* **What the Nurse Can Do to Facilitate These Specific Spiritual/Religious Practices.** When including healer, make time and space for rituals, chants, and prayers. Nurses should not pretend to be familiar with traditions, and should not interfere. Family members would consider it rude to ask a nurse to leave, so be aware and respectful of need for privacy.

BUDDHIST

* **Names by Which the Particular Sect is Known. Buddhist Churches of America, Buddhism.** There are many forms of Buddhism; some sects based on country of origin. As of 1993, there were 554,000 Buddhists in North America.
* **Spiritual/Religious Beliefs That Explain the Presence of Health and Illness.** According to Buddhist tradition, Siddhartha Gautama, the Buddha, who lived in India during 6th century B.C., discovered that this life is basically unsatisfactory when conditioned by a mind full of greed, hatred, and delusion. Unclear mind produces suffering and bad *karma*, leading to repeated rebirths in unsatisfactory worlds. One

transcends this existence through the Eightfold Path: right understanding, right thought, right speech, right action, right livelihood, right effort, right mindfulness, and right concentration. Central focus of most Buddhist practice is attainment of clear, calm state of mind, undisturbed by worldly actions and full of compassion.

Buddhist traditions, beliefs, and levels of commitment vary. Some believe that acts of veneration toward special monks, observing memorial services for ancestors, building temples, chanting, or performing rituals can be as significant for good *karma* as generosity, loving kindness, and compassion from a pure mind.

Illness is a result of *karma* (law of cause an effect); therefore, an inevitable consequence o' actions in this or a previous life. Illness not du to punishment by a divine being. Buddhism teaches way to overcome fears and anxieties. Healing and recovery promoted by awakening to wisdom of Buddha, which results in spiritual peace and freedom from anxiety.

* **Spiritual/Religious Implements.** Incense burning, flower and fruit offerings, altars in temples and home with images of Buddha and ancestors, prayer beads.

* **Daily Practices That Might Be Performed Frequently.** Buddhism does not dictate dogma or any specific practices. Individual differences expected and respected. Individuals may chant or meditate or observe other rites and/or rituals according to form of Buddhism they follow.

* **Food Requirements and Prohibitions.** Extremes are to be avoided. No prescriptions for food; many Buddhists do not eat meat. Buddhism encourages whatever will help individual to attain Enlightenment.

Spiritual/Religious Practices Associated with Life Transitions

* **Pregnancy and Birth.** Artificial insemination, sterility testing, and birth control acceptable. Buddhists do not condone taking a life. Circumstances of patient determine whether abortion acceptable. Birth rites may be observed after child is mature enough.

* **Illness.** Buddhists do not believe in healing through faith. No restrictions on blood or blood products. No religious restrictions on therapy during holy days; consult patient about his/her preferences. Surgical procedures allowed but extremes avoided. If organ donation will help someone else pursue Enlightenment, may be encouraged as act of mercy. If hope for recover and continued pursuit of Enlightenment, all available means of support encouraged.

Buddhists often refrain from using medications, but in great discomfort, medications acceptable as long as they do not affect state of mind (e.g., hallucinations).

* **Dying and Death.** Beliefs based on understanding of impermanence. Enlightenment can be achieved by accepting inevitability of death and opportunity for improvement in next life. Dying person's state of mind at moment of death believed to influence rebirth. Chanting the teachings of Buddha help calm and clear mind. Grief anticipated. Acceptance of death does not mean resignation or refusal of conventional medicine.

    Each Buddhist group has own ritual requirements after death, e.g., last rite chanting at bedside soon after death, family members remaining with body until cremation or burial. Since body considered a shell, autopsy and disposal of body are individual rather than religious decisions although body must be treated with respect. Cremation common and burials usually a brief graveside service after a temple funeral where photograph of deceased may be displayed.

    Pregnant women should avoid funerals to prevent bad luck for baby. Suicide, violent, unexpected death, or death of small child may necessitate monks, soothsayers, or special rituals to counter negative impact of lack of preparation or wrong condition of mind at death.

* **Expected Involvement of Spiritual/Religious Practitioners in the Illness.** Priest or monk may provide counseling or conduct religious rites. Traditions can be carried out by lay community without presence of monk.

* **What the Nurse Can Do to Facilitate These Specific Spiritual/Religious Practices.** Because individual responsibility is acknowledged and many variations of Buddhist practice exist, avoid embarrassment and discomfort by direct discussion of preferences. Ensure calm and peaceful environment and comfort, especially for dying person. Important for family members to be able to say that person died peacefully.

CATHOLIC

* **Names by Which the Particular Sect is Known.** Catholics of the Roman Rite or Roman Catholics are major group among 32 rites comprising Catholicism; membership totals 96 million in North America.

* **Spiritual/Religious Beliefs That Explain the Presence of Health and Illness.** Illness may be God's punishment for sinful thinking or behavior. Suffering is part of one's fate and relates to

religious belief in life after death and eternal victory for the saved. Martyrs are honored.

* **Spiritual/Religious Implements.** Many signs, symbols (especially the name of Jesus Christ, the cross, the crucifix [cross with Jesus' body fixed on it]), music, images, colors, and natural or crafted objects and statues serve as religious implements. Sacred oils and incense used only in official rituals while other implements common in daily life, e.g., candles and holy water. Devotion to saints, particularly Mary, a distinguishing feature of Catholicism, evident in use of images or icons while praying.

* **Daily Practices That Might Be Performed Frequently.** Praying at table, bedtime, or other times, praying the rosary (beads to aid in saying prayers), attending Mass on Sunday, Holy Days and sometimes daily, lighting a candle, blessing with holy water, wearing religious medal or scapular (pieces of cloth), displaying medal or statue for particular intercessional purpose. Symbolic behaviors include gestures (kneeling, genuflecting, prostrating, bowing, striking the breast, folding hands, and raising of hands and eyes, making sign of the cross), rituals and ritual words such as Amen ("So be it"), Alleluia, Hosanna ("Praise the Lord").

* **Food Requirements and Prohibitions.** Use foods in moderation, not injurious to health. Some Catholics abstain from meat on Fridays. At particular times of year, fasting undertaken. Most ill patients exempt from fasting and abstinence.

Spiritual/Religious Practices Associated with Life Transitions

* **Pregnancy and Birth.** Natural means of birth control only. Abortion and sterilization prohibited. Donor insemination and other reproductive technologies may be prohibited. Infant baptism required and urgent if prognosis grave. For all miscarriages, baptism is required. Circumcision permissible.

* **Illness.** Blood and blood products permissible. Medications may be taken if benefits outweigh risks. Organ donation justifiable. Most surgical procedures permissible except abortion and sterilization. A major amputated limb may be buried in consecrated ground. Healing practices include Sacrament of the Sick (which includes anointing, communion if possible, and blessing by a priest), burning candles, laying on of hands, offering prayers. The Eucharist (a wafer of flour and water) may be given as food of healing. Patient also may want Sacrament of Reconciliation (confession).

* **Dying and Death.** Obligated to take ordinary, not extraordinary, means to prolong life. Permissible to refuse treatment that carries risk or would only gain a burdensome prolongation of life. Direct life-ending procedures (euthanasia) forbidden. Sacrament of the Sick mandatory. Autopsy permissible. Organ or body donation justifiable. The body is to be treated with respect. Burial is usual although cremation may be acceptable. Catholic who commits suicide may be denied burial in consecrated ground or Catholic cemetery.

* **Expected Involvement of Spiritual/Religious Practitioners in the Illness.** Father (priest), Mr. or Deacon (deacon), Sister (nun, Catholic woman who has taken vows), Brother (Catholic man who has taken vows) may visit. Any of them, as well as Catholic laypersons, may administer the Eucharist although only Priest can perform Sacrament of the Sick. Catholic Church has many outreach programs for the sick and owns many health care facilities. Catholic Charities and St. Vincent DePaul Society handle serious needs or provide material goods and counseling.

* **What the Nurse Can Do to Facilitate These Specific Spiritual/Religious Practices.** Ask patient and family directly about preferred religious practices and strength of beliefs related to health care. Also ask about preferred religious visitors. Religious representatives will bring necessary supplies for sacraments. Nurse can provide privacy and atmosphere of prayer and quiet. Provide information about patient's ability to swallow and glass of water if patient has difficulty swallowing the Eucharist. Any information that might help religious representative respond more caringly to patient can be provided. Nurse, family members, or other significant people may join in prayer if requested.

CHRISTIAN SCIENTIST

* **Names by Which the Particular Sect is Known.** Church of Christ, Scientist; Christian Science. There are 3000 congregations worldwide.

* **Spiritual/Religious Beliefs That Explain the Presence of Health and Illness.** Christian Science healing starts with Biblical foundation that God created universe and man in perfection. Human imperfections, including all human fears, griefs, wants, sin, emotional disturbance and physical illness, manifest a fundamental misunderstanding of creation. Thus these imperfections can be healed through prayer and spiritual regeneration. Healing occurs as result of drawing closer to God and is

proof of God's care. Faith must not rest on blind belief but on understanding perfection of God's spiritual creation in the present. This differentiates Christian Science from faith healing. Purpose of prayer (Christian Science treatment) is to deal with problems of establishing God's law of harmony in all aspects of life. Physical healing a manifestation of both moral and spiritual change.

Christian Scientists not completely opposed to doctors but may avoid diagnostic testing for fear of being forced to accept unwanted medical treatment in violation of their religious beliefs. Individuals free to make their own decisions in each situation. Most members rely on spiritual healing and believe that true spiritual healing through prayer differs radically from suggestion, will power, and psychotherapy, all of which use human mind as agent of healing.

* **Spiritual/Religious Implements.** Wide variety of books and journals published by Christian Science Publishing Society.
* **Daily Practices That Might Be Performed Frequently.** No outward ceremonies or observances. Deeply meaningful inner experiences include daily sacraments and prayer.
* **Food Requirements and Prohibitions.** No food restrictions. Abstain from alcohol and tobacco. Some abstain from tea and coffee.

Spiritual/Religious Practices Associated with Life Transitions

* **Pregnancy and Birth.** Abortion incompatible with faith. Artificial insemination is unusual. Birth control an individual decision. During childbirth, obstetrician or midwife involved.
* **Illness.** No disease is beyond power of God to heal. Medications, blood and blood products not ordinarily used. Immunizations/vaccines accepted only to comply with law. If limb is lost, might seek a prosthesis. No surgical procedures practiced. Organ donation individual choice but unlikely. Do not seek biopsies or physical examinations. Repair of fractures may be sought. Christian Scientists observe public health requirements for reporting and quarantining individuals with contagious disease.
* **Dying and Death.** Euthanasia contrary to teachings. Unlikely to seek medical help to prolong life. Most do not donate body. Disposal of the body and burial decided by family.
* **Expected Involvement of Spiritual/Religious Practitioners in the Illness.** No clergy. Full-time healing ministers (Christian Science Practitioners) practice spiritual healing and do not use medical or psychological techniques.

Practitioners are lay members of the church and do not conduct public worship services. Visitors include family, friends, and members of Christian Science community, and Christian Science nurses who provide care in facilities or homes. *Christian Science Journal* has a directory of Christian Science nurses available to dress wounds, set bones, and other mechanical healing tasks and provide healing atmosphere. The church operates nursing homes that use spiritual means of health maintenance.

* **What the Nurse Can Do to Facilitate These Specific Spiritual/Religious Practices.** Always clarify whether and to what extent a Christian Scientist and family members are interested in employing medical or psychological techniques/procedures or medications. Advocate for their preference.

HINDU

* **Names by Which the Particular Sect is Known.** Hinduism. Possibly world's oldest religion, evolving over last 4000 years on Indian subcontinent. Founded on sacred, written scripture called *Vedas*. Approximately 1.3 million Hindus in North America.

* **Spiritual/Religious Beliefs That Explain the Presence of Health and Illness.** Vast variety of belief, practices, and customs. No single founder or creed. May be monotheistic, polytheistic, or atheistic. Because there is no universally acceptable scripture or religious hierarchy, ethical code is flexible and subject to local interpretation. *Dharma* is traditional law of morality and ethics that establishes norms and expectations for every part of life and thereby assigns actions and duties to the levels of the caste system. Adherence assures well-being is secured. *Karma* (law of cause and effect) and reincarnation holds a person to actions or duties assigned by *dharma*. Every action has potential for reward or punishment. One cannot change past but present or future actions can modify one's fate over multiple lifetimes. Pain and suffering seen as result of past actions. Future lives influenced by how one faces illness, disability, and/or death. Liberation from cycle of rebirth and re-death is goal of existence. Illness seen as biological, social, and environmental phenomenon. Natural and supernatural causes recognized.

* **Spiritual/Religious Implements.** Some may wear a thread on the torso that should not be removed except in an annual ceremony, or wear a thread around the wrist. People bring offerings to Hindu temples, which are dwellings of deities.

* **Daily Practices That Might Be Performed
  Frequently.** Roles and ceremonies performed
  within framework of caste system, focusing on
  events of birth, marriage, and death. There are
  holy days and many places for religious pilgrimage. Personal hygiene very important and bath
  required every day, but bathing after meal may
  be viewed as injurious. Hot water may be added
  to cold, but not the opposite.

* **Food Requirements and Prohibitions.** Most
  are vegetarians. Wholesome diet emphasized.
  Light meal in morning, heavy meal at midday,
  and another light meal in evening are customary. Hindus venerate life, especially cows.
  According to dietary law, right hand is used for
  eating and left hand for toileting and hygiene.

Spiritual/Religious Practices Associated with Life Transitions

* **Pregnancy and Birth.** Birth control and
  amniocentesis acceptable. No policy on abortion. No restriction on artificial insemination.

* **Illness.** Some people believe in faith healing;
  others that illness is God's punishment for sins.
  Prayer for health considered low form of prayer;
  stoicism preferable. Medications, blood and
  blood products, donation and receipt of organs
  acceptable. Loss of limb (amputation) is due to
  sins of past life.

* **Dying and Death.** Death seen as opposite of
  birth, not opposite of life. Both mark a passage.
  Untimely death mourned because unsatisfied
  karmic debt from past life is carried over to next
  life. One can be consoled by expectation of
  rebirth; therefore, person should be allowed to
  die peacefully. Active euthanasia viewed as
  destructive of *dharma* and producing negative
  karma for those involved. No custom or restriction on prolongation of life although life seen
  as perpetual cycle. Autopsy and organ donation
  acceptable. Before and after death, religious
  prayers and chanting continually offered by
  friends, family, and priests. Men and women
  both very expressive in outward display of grief.
  Rites might include tying a thread around the
  neck or wrist to signify blessing. It is not to be
  removed. Immediately after death, priest may
  pour water into mouth of corpse and family may
  wash the body. Cremation is common; ashes
  disposed of in holy rivers. Fetus or newborn
  may be buried.

* **Expected Involvement of Spiritual/Religious
  Practitioners in the Illness.** Religious practitioner is priest. Priesthood achieved through
  reincarnation; priests greatly respected but
  unlikely to be involved in illness care.
  Minimal formal organization and no religious

organizations to help the sick. Help provided by significant others within the caste.

*   **What the Nurse Can Do to Facilitate These Specific Spiritual/Religious Practices.** Question patient and family about what practices are important to them and, to degree possible, create environment to facilitate these practices. Ask about beliefs about folk medicine and guard against conflict with these practices unless they could be harmful. Involve family members in plan of care and determine which member will provide personal care. Father/husband is primary spokesperson to whom questions should be directed to gain his trust so that nurse no longer seen as intruder. After death, communicate respect by providing privacy for family to carry out rites.

ISLAM

*   **Names by Which the Particular Sect is Known.** Islam, a word meaning peace or complete submission, is name of monotheistic religion preached by Prophet Mohammed around Mecca approximately 1,400 years ago. Musselman, Muslim, or Moslem are names given to people who profess Islamic faith. There are 2.6 million Muslims in U.S.

*   **Spiritual/Religious Beliefs That Explain the Presence of Health and Illness.** Belief in only one God, or *Allah*, is most important principle in Islam. Other guiding principles are: to believe in Prophet Mohammed and Holy *Koran*; to believe there is a judgment day and life after death; to make a commitment to fast; *haj*, to go at least once, if possible, on pilgrimage to Mecca; *zakat*, to perform duty to give with generosity to poor people; *jihad*, to fight for sake of *Allah*; and to pray five times each day. Principal object of faith to show the straight path by which people's faculties are brought to perfection and individual souls may experience full self-realization. The law of an Islamic state is the law of the *Koran*. Since life is gift of God, disease, pain and suffering are manifestations of God's will. Pain and suffering part of expiating sin.

*   **Spiritual/Religious Implements.** Holy *Koran* (word of God) and *hadith* (traditional sayings and acts of Prophet Mohammed). Patient may wear chain with symbol of Islam, use prayer rug, or wear a *taawiz* (*Koranic* verses wrapped in a small cloth).

*   **Daily Practices That Might be Performed Frequently.** Prayer five times a day facing Mecca, after ritual washing (dawn, mid-day, mid-afternoon, sunset, nightfall). Days of

observance occur throughout Muslim lunar calendar. No sacraments.

*   **Food Requirements and Prohibitions.** Pork, alcohol, and some shellfish prohibited. Moderation expected. During *Ramadan* (*Ramazan* among Farsi speakers) (ninth month), daylight fasting (including fluids) practiced. Children, pregnant women and those in fragile physical condition exempt.

Spiritual/Religious Practices Associated with Life Transitions

*   **Pregnancy and Birth.** Birth control acceptable. Religious objections to abortion. Artificial insemination permitted between husband and wife. Before 130 days, aborted fetus discarded as any other tissue, but after 130 days, considered full human being. Circumcision of male children before five years of age. Although not a religious requirement, some Moslems from Africa, the Middle East, Indonesia, Malaysia, and India practice female circumcision, usually when the girl is young.
*   **Illness.** No restrictions on blood or blood products. Faith healing generally not acceptable unless done to prevent deterioration of patient's psychological condition and morale. For some, use of herbal remedies and faith healing practiced. Medications, blood, blood products, amputations, organ transplants, and biopsies not restricted. Most surgical procedures permitted. Older or conservative Muslims may not readily adhere to therapy because of fatalistic view.
*   **Dying and Death.** Euthanasia or any attempt to shorten life prohibited. Right to die not accepted. Organ or body donations acceptable. Autopsy only permitted for medical or legal reasons although devout people may be concerned about desecration of human body. Confession of sins and begging forgiveness must occur in presence of family before death. Important to follow five steps of burial procedure which specifies washing, dressing, and positioning of the body. First step is traditional washing of the body by Muslim of same gender.
*   **Expected Involvement of Spiritual/Religious Practitioners in the Illness.** Family and friends visit to provide emotional and financial support. No specific church organizations to help the sick.
*   **What the Nurse Can Do to Facilitate These Specific Spiritual/Religious Practices.** Explore with patient and family what beliefs and practices are most significant to them. Provide environment conducive to carrying out these practices.

JEHOVAH'S WITNESS

* **Names by Which the Particular Sect is Known.** Jehovah's Witnesses, Watch Tower Bible and Tract Society. North American membership approximately 1.5 million. Name of Jehovah's Witnesses comes from Hebrew name for "God" (Jehovah) in the King James Bible.

* **Spiritual/Religious Beliefs That Explain the Presence of Health and Illness.** Opposition to "false teachings" of other sects, often extending to science and medicine. Conversion of others important. Ten hours or more every month devoted to proselytizing activities. Some are conscientious objectors in war. Do not participate in nationalistic ceremonies (e.g., saluting the flag) or give gifts at holidays nor do they celebrate traditional Christian holy days. Give full allegiance to Jehovah's kingdom. Believe that after world has been restored to state of paradise, beneficiaries of Christ will be resurrected with healthy, perfected physical bodies and will inhabit earth.

* **Spiritual/Religious Implements.** Bible; no sacraments.

* **Daily Practices That Might Be Performed Frequently.** Prayer and reading of scriptures.

* **Food Requirements and Prohibitions.** Abstain from tobacco. Moderate use of alcohol, but drunkenness a sin.

Spiritual/Religious Practices Associated with Life Transitions

* **Pregnancy and Birth.** Abortion, artificial insemination, and sterilization forbidden. Other birth control methods individual choice. No infant baptism.

* **Illness.** Faith healing forbidden. Reading scriptures believed to comfort individual and lead to mental and spiritual healing. Medications accepted unless derived from blood products. Strongly opposed to blood transfusion. Prohibition of blood based on scripture and Christian history. Blood volume expanders acceptable if not derived from blood. Devices for circulating blood acceptable if not primed with blood. Surgical procedures not opposed per se but administration of blood products completely prohibited. Some hospitals and physicians have turned to the courts to mandate treatment involving blood. Organ transplants may be forbidden if bodily mutilation occurs. Use of extraordinary means to prolong life or right to die is individual choice.

* **Dying and Death.** Euthanasia forbidden. Autopsy acceptable if legally required. No last rites. Donation of the body or organs forbidden.

Burial determined by individual preference and local custom.

* **Expected Involvement of Spiritual/Religious Practitioners in the Illness.** Members of congregation and elders visit to pray for sick person and read scriptures.
* **What the Nurse Can Do to Facilitate These Specific Spiritual/Religious Practices.** Remain sensitive to strong religious beliefs underlying opposition to use of blood or other controversial health care issues. Determine strength of patient's and family's beliefs, especially regarding blood products. Act as patient advocate and provide support. Provide privacy and quiet for prayer and scripture reading.

JEWISH

* **Names by Which the Particular Sect is Known.** Judaism, Jews. Judaism is an Old Testament monotheistic religion dating back to Prophet Abraham. Approximately 7 million Jews in U.S. in three major groups: Orthodox, Conservative, and Reform. Hasidic Jews, a fundamentalist sect, live mainly in Eastern metropolitan areas.
* **Spiritual/Religious Beliefs That Explain the Presence of Health and Illness.** Historically, Jewish law contained in the *Torah* and explained orally and in the *Talmud* prescribed most daily actions of people. In Judaism, commitments, obligations, duties, and commandments have priority over rights and individual pleasures. Illness may occur as punishment for sin. In case of illness, medical care from physician expected according to Jewish law. Jews have strong belief in sanctity of life. Each situation of health care decision making must be considered individually on its own merits with assistance of rabbi.
* **Spiritual/Religious Implements.** Strictly observant male patient may put on prayer shawl, *yarmulka* (cap), and *tfillin* (look like black strings) tied onto arms and forehead while praying.
* **Daily Practices that Might Be Performed Frequently.** Orthodox and Conservative Jews observe Sabbath from sundown Friday to sundown Saturday. Orthodox Jews may refrain from all forms of work, including using machinery, cars, and cooking, during Sabbath. There are 13 other holy days special to practicing Jews. Unless rabbi counsels that surgical procedure is necessary and therefore permitted by Talmudic law, Jews may avoid procedures during these days. Preservation of life highest priority and main criterion for determining activities on holy days.

* **Food Requirements and Prohibitions.**
Orthodox Jews and some Conservative Jews
observe strict dietary laws: milk and meat not
mixed or eaten together and separate cookware
and utensils used. Predatory fowl, shellfish, and
pork products forbidden. Of water creatures,
only fish with fins and scales permissible.
Complex rules regarding food preparation. May
request *kosher* (which actually means "properly
prepared") products only. Reform Jews rarely
observe kosher dietary laws. Wine a part of religious observance and guideline is moderation.

Spiritual/Religious Practices Associated with Life Transitions

* **Pregnancy and Birth.** Considered a good deed
to have children. Therapeutic abortion permitted. Within some groups, abortion on demand
is accepted but not as method of birth control.
Aborted fetus considered a potential human
being and is buried, not discarded. Artificial
insemination permitted but rabbi must be consulted in each case. Birth control permitted,
except with Orthodox Jews. Ritual circumcision
(*Bris*) of males mandatory among Orthodox
and Conservative Jews on eighth day of life.
Reform Jews favor but do not require ritual
circumcision.

* **Illness.** Medical care expected. No restrictions
on medications. Judaism prohibits ingesting
blood but this is not applicable to transfusions.
Organ donation a complex issue (see below).
Most surgical procedures allowed. Amputated
or surgically removed body parts should be
available to family for burial.

* **Dying and Death.** Euthanasia prohibited.
Autopsy permitted when legally required. All
body parts must be buried together, never
donated or removed. People have right to die
with dignity; ongoing procedures must be continued but no new procedures need to be undertaken. When death imminent and all medical
options are exhausted, Judaism does not mandate use of life-prolonging measures. The body
may be ritually washed after death by members
of Ritual Burial Society. Cosmetic restoration or
efforts to change pace of natural decomposition
(embalming) discouraged. Burial should take
place as soon as possible. Cremation not appropriate. Mourning extends over a year and
includes practices that influence all aspects of
life including an initial 7-day period of mourning called *shiva.*

* **Expected Involvement of Spiritual/Religious
Practitioners in the Illness.** In Jewish liturgy
there are many prayers for the sick (which may
be chanted) and hope for recovery. Visit from

rabbi may be spent talking or praying with patient alone or with a group of ten adults. Other visitors include family and friends from synagogue. Many community services, such as Jewish Federation and Jewish Community Service, available for variety of needs.

* **What the Nurse Can Do to Facilitate These Specific Spiritual/Religious Practices.** Discuss patient's expected observance of any holy days occurring during hospital stay or need for spiritual implements. Find out if patient wants kosher food and whether patient is referring to type of food or how food is prepared. Provide privacy for visits with rabbi and for prayer/chanting. Hasidic Jews have very specific beliefs and practices that must be considered in provision of health care (such as patients not being touched by care providers of opposite gender). Explore in detail specific expectations or requirements and make necessary adjustments in planning care.

MORMON

* **Names by Which the Particular Sect is Known.** Church of Jesus Christ of Latter Day Saints (LDS), Mormonism. North American membership 6.5 million.
* **Spiritual/Religious Beliefs That Explain the Presence of Health and Illness.** One of central purposes of life is procreation. Power of God can be exercised to bring healing of illness. Faith healing (faith in Jesus Christ and power of priesthood to heal) and medical care/treatment used together. Medical intervention viewed as one of God's ways of using humans to heal. Mormons believe that life continues beyond death.
* **Spiritual/Religious Implements.** After being considered worthy to enter a temple, Mormon wears a type of underclothing called a garment which signifies promises to God. Garment may be removed for care although older people may not want to give it up in hospital. Blessing of sick uses consecrated oil.
* **Daily Practices that Might Be Performed Frequently.** Sacrament meetings are held on Sunday which is Sabbath in U.S. Sacraments called ordinances. Some occur only in temples. Baptism at 8 years old or after, never during infancy or at death.
* **Food Requirements and Prohibitions.** Alcohol, tobacco, coffee, and tea prohibited. There is counsel against but not prohibition of caffeine-containing soft drinks. Fasting (no food or drink for 24 hours) required once each month. Ill people are not required to fast.

Spiritual/Religious Practices Associated with Life Transitions

*   **Pregnancy and Birth.** Birth control contrary to Mormon belief. Abortion forbidden except when mother's life is in danger or woman chooses to abort pregnancy resulting from rape. Artificial insemination acceptable between husband and wife.
*   **Illness.** No restrictions on blood or blood products or medications. May use herbal folk remedies. Organ donation permitted. Surgical procedures an individual decision. Healing practices include blessing of the sick which consists of two Elders anointing with oil, sealing the anointing with prayer and blessing, and laying hands on head of patient.
*   **Dying and Death.** Euthanasia not practiced because people must not interfere with God's plan. Promote peaceful and dignified death if death inevitable. Organ donation an individual choice. With consent of next of kin, autopsy permitted. Burial in "temple clothes" usual custom.
*   **Expected Involvement of Spiritual/Religious Practitioners in the Illness.** When performing blessing of the sick, Elders will bring vial of consecrated oil and if performing Sacrament of the Lord's Supper, will bring what is needed. Visitors include strong network of church members (Elder, Sister and other representatives), family and friends. Members helped by the Relief Society.
*   **What the Nurse Can Do to Facilitate These Specific Spiritual/Religious Practices.** Ask about use of herbal remedies. Allow for visits by church representatives. Provide privacy and quiet for sacraments. Always ask patient and family about specific preferences.

PROTESTANT

*   **Names by Which the Particular Sect is Known.** Many Christian groups in U.S., including 30 Baptist denominations, Christian Church (also Disciples of Christ, Churches of Christ), Episcopal (also Anglican), Lutheran (4 groups), Mennonites (also Hutterites and Amish), United Methodist Church, Reformed-Presbyterian, Presbyterian, Unitarian Universalist Association, and United Church of Christ (Congregational Church, Christian Church, Evangelical synod, and Reformed church).
*   **Spiritual/Religious Beliefs That Explain the Presence of Health and Illness.** Within many traditions and groups, varied beliefs about health and illness. Protestants generally

emphasize individual responsibility and conscience over following tradition or religious authority.

*   **Spiritual/Religious Implements.** Bible.
*   **Daily Practices That Might Be Performed Frequently.** Prayer. Additional practices may be appropriate on Holy Days (as defined within each denomination).
*   **Food Requirements and Prohibitions.** Individual choice. Alcohol and drugs may be proscribed in more fundamentalist groups.

Spiritual/Religious Practices Associated with Life Transitions

*   **Pregnancy and Birth.** In most denominations, decisions about genetic counseling, birth control, sterility tests, and artificial insemination are individual decisions. In some denominations, there are restrictions. Baptism may be practiced, sometimes by immersion, often after infancy.
*   **Illness.** In most denominations, decisions about blood, blood products, vaccines, biopsies, amputations, and transplants are individual. Prayer, reading scripture, taking of communion, fasting, "laying on of hands," anointing with oil, and/or anointing and blessing of the sick may be practiced in health crisis.
*   **Dying and Death.** Organ donation, autopsy, and burial or cremation usually individual decisions. Prolonging life (right to die) may have restrictions. With regard to euthanasia, positions vary from individual decision to religious restriction. Many groups prohibit euthanasia based on belief that only God gives life and only God can take it (Lutheran, Mennonite); discuss with family, patient and representative of church. Episcopal and Lutheran may allow for termination of extraordinary treatment but not active euthanasia. Others emphasize value of life but do not regard active euthanasia as inconsistent with this respect (Reformed-Presbyterian, United Church of Christ). Unitarian Universalists provide denominational support for euthanasia.
*   **Expected Involvement of Spiritual/Religious Practitioners in the Illness.** Personal choice of patient and family. Visits of clergy for counsel and prayer frequently helpful.
*   **What the Nurse Can Do to Facilitate These Specific Spiritual/Religious Practices.** Ask patient and family what practices would provide support to them and create an environment conducive to these practices.

APPENDIX B

Selected References

Andrews, M. M., & Boyle, J. S. (1995). *Transcultural concepts in nursing care* (2nd ed.). Philadelphia: J.B. Lippincott.

Beliefs that can affect therapy. (1975). *Nursing update.* Darien, CT: Miller & Fink Corp.

Dues, G. (1989). *Catholic customs & traditions: A popular guide.* Mystic, CT: Twenty-third Publications.

Gigar, J. N., & Davidhizar, R. E. (1991). *Transcultural nursing: Assessment and intervention.* St. Louis: Mosby Year Book.

Hamel, R., & DuBose, E. R. (1991). Part four: Views of the major faith traditions. *In Active euthanasia, religion, and the public debate.* Chicago: The Park Ridge Center.

Irish, D. P., Lundquist, K. F., & Nelsen, V. J. (1993). *Ethnic variations in dying, death, and grief: Diversity in universality.* Washington, DC: Taylor & Francis, Inc.

May, L. (1995). Challenging medical authority: The refusal of treatment by Christian Scientists. *Hastings Center Report, 25*(1), 15-21.

McGoldrick, M., Pearce, J. K., & Giordano, J. (1982). *Ethnicity and family therapy.* NY: Guilford.

Rispler-Chaim, V. (1993). The ethics of postmortem examinations in contemporary Islam. *Journal of Medical Ethics 19,* 164-168.

Shaw, E. (1985). Female circumcision. *American Journal of Nursing, 85*(6), 684-687.

Spector, R. E. (1991). *Cultural diversity in health and illness* (3rd ed.). Norwalk, CT: Appleton & Lange.

Steinberg, A. (1994). The terminally ill—secular and Jewish ethical aspects. *Israel Journal of Medical Science, 30,* 130-135.

Stover, D. (1996). Native healing practices. In P. D. Barry (Ed.), *Psychosocial nursing: Care of physically ill patients and their families* (3rd ed.) (pp. 67, 72). Philadelphia: Lippincott.

Zumbro Valley Medical Society, Medicine and Religion Committee. (1978). *Religious aspects of medical care: A handbook of religious practices of all faiths* (2nd Ed.). St. Louis: The Catholic Hospital Association.

APPENDIX C

Selected Regions of the World Maps

ASIA

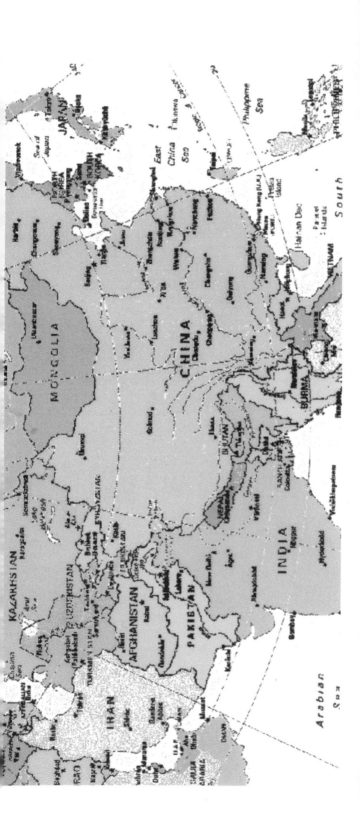

LATIN AMERICA

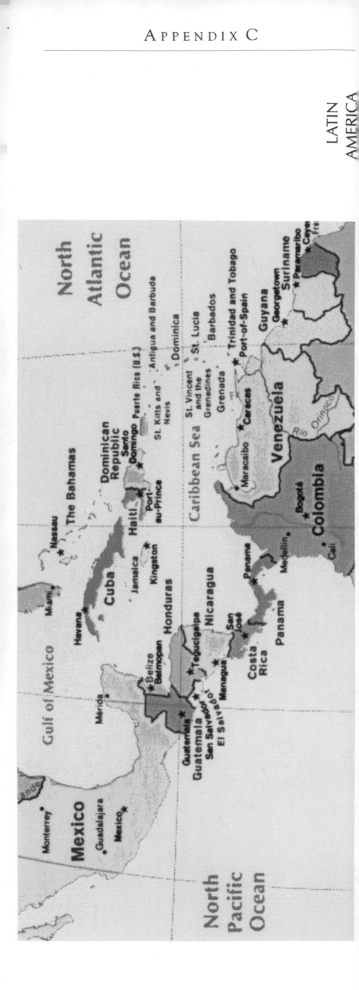

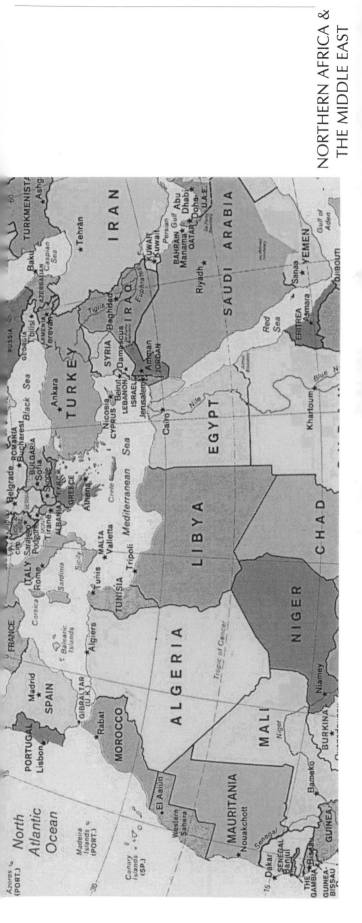

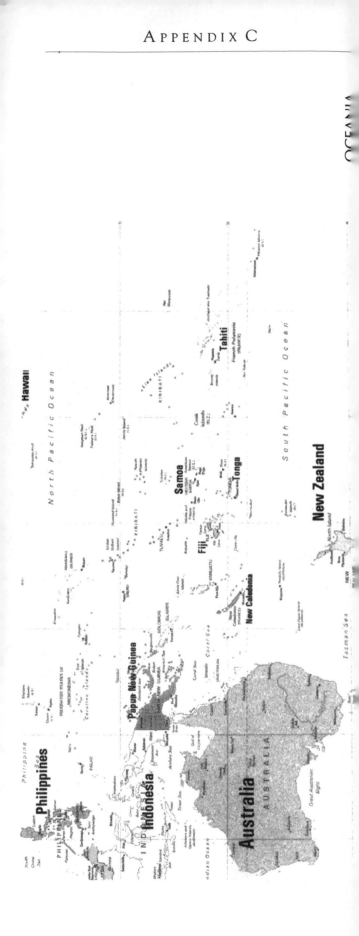

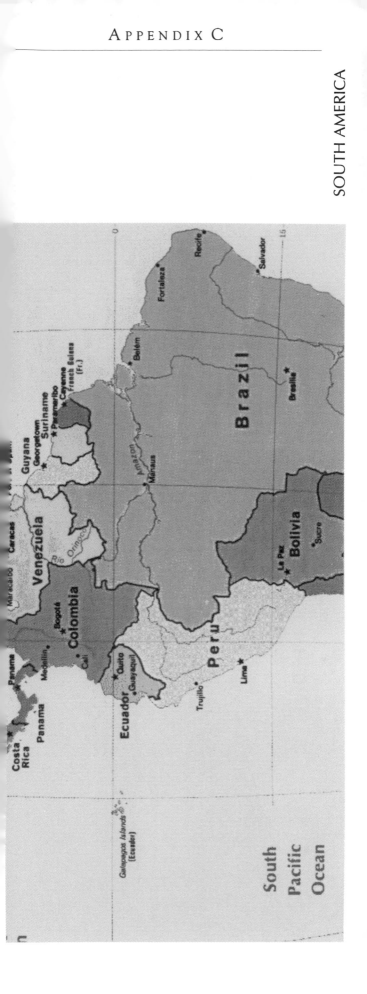

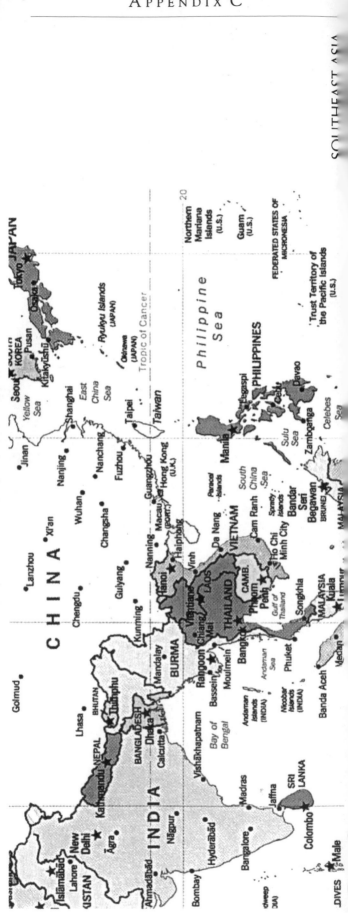